COMMIT TO BE FIT:
Now and Forever

Steve Frierman
Hofstra University

American Press
Boston, Massachusetts
www.americanpresspublishsers.com

Dedication

I am dedicating this book to my family and friends. Tracy, Josh and Jeremy—you have always been there to listen to me over and over again. The three of you have challenged me to conquer new and exciting horizons both personally and professionally which would not have been possible without your love and belief in me. Mom and Dad, you have taught me to always believe in myself no matter how demanding life became. Mindy and Linda, your guidance and strength (using opposite approaches of course) to always look after me and allow me to express myself in a manner that only you two could understand. Arlene (Mom #2)—for your generosity and passion to help me complete this project; Adam, for allowing me to overload your listening skills and let me talk and talk ... you have taught me the meaning of what a true friend is all about. Last but certainly not least, Marc, thanks bro, this one's for you.

Acknowledgements

Somewhere along the line in writing this book, I realized that I could not do it all by myself (what a startling revelation). Sure, I could handle the writing, but the downloading and labeling of the pictures, sending it out, getting the consent forms together, complying with self-imposed deadlines, needing quiet in a house with a Type A wife, two growing boys and two nervous dogs, staying on task with my classes and making sure to find the time to exercise, could not have happened without the help of the following people:

Blake—thanks for labeling the pictures and always making sure that everything got done. In addition to helping me in my office, you have helped me in my life, too. Josh—the master picture taker, if only you knew how to download, too; you're a role model to stay behind the scenes; Jem—among your many talents, you always listened to me and helped me get through some of the tough times; Frankels—having you in my life is like winning the lottery; you're one in a million, make than 10 million; Wolfs—the warmth and generosity that you have given me makes me speechless (and you know that is not an easy task for me); Min—you've taught me many things in life, now it's my turn, read the book, chapter 1 is due on the 29th; Katie, Adam, Kirsten, Dan J., Dan S., Mike, Andrew, Lisa, Jaclyn, Stephanie, Nick, Jessica Rachel, Dara and Josh—thanks for taking part in the picture process; My students and personal training clients—you have revitalized my skills by consistently challenging me to find ways to teach you how to improve your fitness and love the process NOW AND FOREVER. I thank you all; The faculty and staff in the PESP department—thanks for showing an interest in my accomplishments; we make a great team; Finally, Marcie, you invited my style and creativeness and allowed me to express myself in a way that I will always appreciate. I thank you all!

Preface

About three years ago I was presenting at a conference in Albuquerque, New Mexico and then reviewing a rough draft of the chapters I had written for this book. I thought to myself, "Wow, this is great stuff. In fact, it's what you've been teaching people for years. How come you don't do it consistently in your own life?" Then it dawned on me. How could I educate others how to be fit and stay fit if I do not utilize the same concepts and principles to meet my own health-related fitness needs? It was at that point in my life that I had a huge breakthrough. "It's time you practice what you preach." If I know what works for others then I should apply this information to myself and reap the benefits. I decided to go for a jog and rather than overwork myself by trying to get months of fitness back in one run, I simply slowed down, enjoyed the sites and praised myself for my effort to simply get started. What a first for me! Today, I am proud to say that I have consistently kept up with my fitness. I have run in several races ranging from a 5K to a half marathon. I have consistently placed in the top 10-20 percent, running faster and longer than I ever have in my entire life. In addition, my wife and I go the gym to lift together on a regular basis, supporting and encouraging each other and most of all having fun together.

For the past 18 years, I have developed, modified and taught a variety of courses in higher education emphasizing health-related fitness in the following capacity (assessment, prescription, improvement, personal training, motivation). I have had the pleasure (most of the time) of teaching over 2000 students how to exercise properly and have fun in the process. Most recently, I have expanded my horizons to conduct one on one personal training sessions with middle-aged clients. My goal has and continues to be to find ways to motivate individuals to be fit and stay fit for ever. As much as I have taught my students and clients, I have learned at least as much as they have, if not more. Specifically, I have learned that regardless of how much people know about the importance of exercise, they are not going to make exercise part of their lives unless they are committed to living healthy and enjoy the hard work necessary to achieve desirable results.

Now it is your turn to your learn. Learn what motivates you to exercise, what stops you from being more physically active and the strategies to overcome your exercise barriers. Learn how to set goals that motivate you to work hard and feel good about yourself in the process. Most important, learn how to become committed to be fit: now and forever. Below is an outline of each chapter. I bet you can't wait to get started reading!

Chapter 1 begins by introducing the barriers that stop people from being more physically active and fit. Discover what may be stopping you from not exercising enough or even at all (even though you know you could and should). In chapter 2, you will uncover the various motives you have to exercise. You will discover which motive(s) work best for you to begin and eventually continue exercising for a lifetime. Chapter 3 enlightens you on the purposes of setting goals and introduces you to two of the most effective ways to set goals: (1) BE SMAART and (2) Stairway to Success. You will identify some of the problems that may occur when setting goals and then apply several strategies designed to minimize and ultimately prevent them from occurring in the future. This will help you to improve three crucial factors related to long-term exercise participation: (1) enjoyment; (2) performance and (3) commitment to continue. In chapter 4, eight basic principles of lifetime fitness are introduced in order to teach you the guidelines of how to improve your fitness and exercise properly. After being introduced to each principle, you will be asked several questions that help you to apply each principle towards meeting your own individual fitness needs. Chapter 5 addresses seven important questions to help you determine your desire to exercise. By answering these questions, you will begin to learn exactly how committed you are toward exercise while you establish a "Plan" for how to fit exercise into your life.

Chapter 6 begins by introducing you to cardiorespiratory endurance (CRE). Learn why CRE is so important to living healthy. Discover how to formally and informally assess your CRE and learn how to develop a personalized exercise prescription for CRE based on your own level of CR fitness as well as your level of commitment to improve. Find out how to set SMAART goals designed to increase your CRE fitness, enjoyment and motivation. Learn how to prevent injuries and evaluate the success of your CRE program as the weeks go by. In chapter 7, you will differentiate muscular strength from muscular endurance and learn how to develop exercise prescriptions for each. Determine the benefits of working on muscular fitness and when you should increase or decrease weight, reps, sets and exercises. Identify ways to spice up your program to create new and inviting challenges. Programs are included for three levels of muscular fitness (beginner-intermediate-advanced) as well as three levels of commitment (low-moderate-high). Chapter 8 focuses on flexibility where you will learn what flexibility is, the benefits of being flexible and how to develop your own exercise prescription for flexibility. You will be introduced to four different flexibility training techniques: (1) static, (2) passive static, (3) ballistic and (4) PNF. Strengths and limitations of each approach will be discussed and programs will be included for three levels of flexibility (beginner, intermediate-advanced as well commitment (low-moderate-high). In chapter 9, you will distinguish the differences between poor vs. healthy eating. Recognize why people eat poorly; compare the old vs. new food guide pyramids; find out about the six basic nutrients; determine your own daily nutritional intake; discover how committed you are to eat healthier and learn strategies to improve your eating habits; set SMAART goals to improve your nutritional habits and evaluate the success of your eating habits over time;

Chapter 10 introduces you to a variety of different ways to assess body composition. You will learn the differences between being underweight, overweight, over-fat and obese. Discover strategies to improve body composition and determine exactly how committed you are to improving your own body composition. In chapter 11, you will be introduced to four different cognitive strategies (association, dissociation, positive self-talk and imagery. Each strategy is designed to help you take control of your thoughts and maximize thinking while exercising. You will practice each of the four different cognitive strategies and then evaluate the effectiveness of each in enhancing your enjoyment, motivation, performance and commitment to continue exercising. In the final chapter 12, you will discover what stress is and then identify the stressors in your life. You will find out how to take control of your stress by incorporating five different stress management techniques: (1) progressive muscle relaxation; (2) relaxation response; (3) yogic breathing); (4) time out and (5) exercise; Finally, you will evaluate the success of each in decreasing your distress and increasing your eustress.

So there you have it: 12 exciting and invigorating chapters just waiting for you to read and apply in your life. My goal for you is that after reading this book you will have a high level of commitment to exercise and you will have transformed "working out and living healthy" from something you should do to something you do simply because living healthy is part of who you have become. So, commit to be fit: now and forever (what a catchy title)!

Contents

9   EATING HEALTHY

10   BODY COMPOSITION

Chapter 1

What's Stopping You?

In this chapter you will:

- Identify what stops you from being more physically active
- Determine what really motivates you to be more physically active
- Prepare yourself to get started exercising

Each year more and more people are recognizing the importance of living a healthy lifestyle. Factors such as medical doctors recommending and prescribing physical activity and exercise to treat and promote mental and physical health, healthier lifestyles and longevity, business corporations making monetary contributions to local exercise facilities for employee membership and an increase in exercise programs in both public and private sectors have increased the knowledge about the importance of exercising, eating properly and living healthier in youth, adult, and elderly populations.

Unfortunately, knowledge about the importance of exercise and how to exercise properly has not been enough to keep most people physically active and exercising for long periods of time. Over the years, research has discovered that only 20% of the North American population exercises enough to achieve cardiovascular benefits. Approximately 40% are active to a lesser degree, with some receiving health-related benefits, and at least 40% are completely sedentary. Further research has demonstrated that over half the population in North America who begin an exercise program quit within the first six months (Wankel, 1987). More recently, the U.S. Department of Health and Human Services (USDHHS) reported that only one of the 13 physical activity and fitness objectives proposed by the federal government's Healthy People 2000 document was actually met (USDHHS, 2004).

THE QUESTION IS WHY?

Why is that most people know how to live healthy and for the most part be more physically active and eat right, yet we choose not to. Although at one time it was thought that a lack of activity was due to a complete lack of motivation, today researchers have discovered a variety of reasons, referred to as "barriers," that interfere with the motivation to become more physically active and exercising on a regular basis. In this chapter, you will identify the barriers that stop you from being more physically active and discover what motivates you to become more physically active and fit. So let's get started.

WHAT'S STOPPING YOU?

If you think you would like to be more physically active and live a healthier lifestyle, but you haven't yet incorporated physical activity or exercise into your daily routine, why haven't you been doing it? Obviously, something is stopping you and /or motivating you more strongly not to exercise. In order to get started exercising again, you must first examine what is stopping you. Take a few moments and answer the following questions:

1. When was the last time you were physically active?
2. How long did you keep it up for (days, weeks, months)?
3. When did you stop?
4. Why do you think you stopped?

If you are like most people, your answer(s) to question 4 will probably parallel at least one or most of these eight common reasons: (1) I didn't have time; (2) I didn't enjoy it; (3) I didn't get the results I wanted; (4) I didn't have a good place to exercise; (5) I didn't have anyone to show me how to exercise correctly; (6) I couldn't reach my own goals; (7) I injured myself and just never got back to it; (8) My significant other didn't support my efforts.

While many individuals are confronted with these exercise barriers, only a small percentage, approximately 20% have been able to overcome them and stay physically active for a lifetime. The rest of you get stopped and allow these barriers to take control of your lives.

Everyone who is involved in exercise, whether it is contemplating when to start exercising or exercising on a regular basis has been confronted with barriers that may stop that from action. Imagine for a moment if you actually knew what might stop you from exercising before you actually quit. Now imagine if you had access to strategies that could remove these barriers and teach you how to fit exercise into your life without stopping. Well, don't fret—by the time you complete this book, you will be there—exercising on a regular basis and loving every minute of it. So let's find out what may be stopping you.

IDENTIFYING YOUR EXERCISE BARRIERS

No time—This is the most popular reason people give for not exercising (Lox, Martin Ginis, & Petruzzello, 2006; Gettman, Pollock, & Ward, 1983). While phrases like "I would if I had the time" or "I'm so busy" imply that you would exercise if only the time was right or there was more time in the day, this is really more of a perception than a reality (Willis & Campbell, 1992). In fact, if you take a closer look into your daily schedule, how much time do you make to watch television, talk on the phone, read the newspaper, answer your e-mail and surf the web? If you have time for any of that, then you certainly have time to exercise. The question becomes not whether or not you have time to exercise, but do you really want to make the time to exercise?

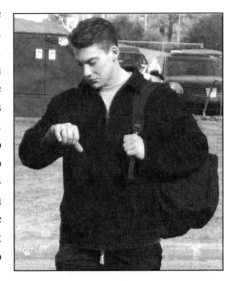

"Where did the time go?"

Ironically, research has shown that people who exercise regularly accomplish more in their day than people who don't (Thayer, 2001; Shaw, Bonen, & McAbe, 1991). Now take a few moments and think about a time in your life when you exercised regularly and compare it with a time that you were less physically active. Do you notice a difference in the amount of energy that you had? What about your productivity at school or work? Did you feel more energetic and productive because you chose not to exercise or because you did exercise? Did you ever not have the time to do what you wanted because of exercising?

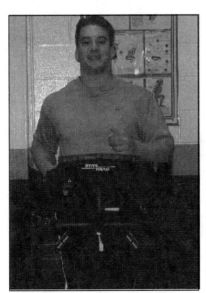

"I found the time to exercise."

If you are like most people then you probably noticed you felt more invigorated and full of energy after exercising and tired and lethargic during the times in your life that you weren't exercising. Scientists have explained that when we exercise, our endorphins (which are a morphine-like substance) are released from the pituitary gland in the brain and induce feelings of euphoria and well-being. This gives you more energy to be productive and accomplish more in a day than if we didn't exercise.

Once you learn how to make exercise a priority in your life, you will find the time. Oh sure, sometimes you may have to modify your exercise schedule, but you will inevitably find the time for the things that provide you the most benefits (e.g. better health, more energy, greater productivity at work, having fun, happier moods, less stress) that lead to a higher quality of life.

So the next time you tell yourself that you can't exercise because you don't have the time—think again. Do you really not have the time or do you not want to make the time? Remember, there are 1440 minutes in every day and all you need is about 2% (20-30 minutes) of that per day to exercise and reap all the benefits of living and being healthy.

No fun—Another popular reason people give for not exercising is that it is "no fun." To put it simply, if you don't enjoy exercising, then why would you want to find the time to do it? While many people give reasons such as: "I want to lose weight"; "I want to tone my muscles"; or "My doctor said I had to" the bottom line is if you're not having fun exercising, you're not going to do it over the long term (Franklin, 1986; Emmons & Diener, 1986). You may make the initial effort to get started, but before long, you will start focusing on all the reasons not to do it. Later in the book, you will identify the things in your life that you perceive to be fun and then learn how to incorporate these activities into your exercise routine.

Lack of results—If you start working out and don't achieve the results that you are seeking, you are probably going to quit exercising. After all, why put in "hard time" if you are not getting what you want out of it. Problems such as setting unrealistic goals (e.g., lose 10 lbs in the next two weeks), being misinformed by exercise infomercials (e.g., turn fat into muscle), overemphasizing physiological factors (e.g., washboard abs; increasing muscular size in a few short workouts) and exercising improperly are just a few of the reasons why people sense of lack of accomplishment, become impatient and look to quit exercising. Unfortunately, nothing that you truly have a passion to achieve is possible without hard work and dedication. So before you even start your workout, you should make sure that the results you want are reasonable, attainable and 100% within your control. (Chapter 3 entitled "BE SMAART" helps you set important goals that are focused on getting the results that you want both in the short and long term).

Inconvenient Location/Convenience—Having to travel far distances, inaccessible transportation, lack of facilities, and poor or lack of equipment are just a few of the more popular reasons why people fail to engage in regular physical activity (Lox, Martin Ginis, & Petruzzello, 2006). Research has demonstrated that proximity and convenience to the exercise facility were two of the most important factors in exercise participation for both corporate and community exercise programs (Teraslinna, Partanen, Koskela, & Oja, 1969; Cox, 1984; Goodrick, Hartung, Warren, & Hoepfel, 1984). In fact, the easier the facility is to get to, the better your chances of using it. So for those of you who have extra space in your house, why not see about getting some exercise equipment. For those of you who work in large corporations, consider asking your boss about having an exercise facility on or near the office. Research has found that effectively run corporate fitness programs have increased employee productivity, improved efficiency, concentration, creativity, and decision making time, increased morale, reduced mental errors and worker absenteeism, decreased health care, disability, and worker compensation costs, and reduced employee turnover (Genesis Personal fitness: Your 1st step is to begin http://www.genesis personal/fitness.com/CorporateFitness.htm) Just tell your boss that a fit worker is a more productive worker.

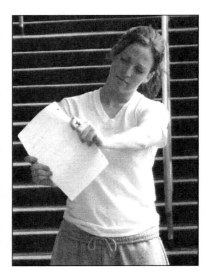

Poor exercise leader—Perhaps the most important determinant of an individual's continued participation in an exercise program is the quality of leadership (Franklin, 1988, Weinberg & Gould, 2007). A good exercise leader is someone who has a positive influence on exercisers and can contribute to increases in their fitness, self-efficacy, enjoyment, and motivation to exercise. A good exercise leader should be energetic and enthusiastic and can identify and meet the needs of their exercisers. He/she should have a formal education in the exercise sciences (e.g., exercise physiology, exercise psychology, health-related fitness, counseling, personal training) and have expertise in creating a safe exercise environment, developing proper exercise prescriptions and motivating clients to exercise on their own. In contrast, the poor exercise leader is someone who can have a negative social influence on exercisers and may ultimately cause them to drop out of a fitness program (Lox, Martin-Ginis, & Petruzzello, 2006; Bray, Gyurcsik,, Culos-Reed, Dawson, & Martin, 2001). He/she often uses criticism and blame rather than praise and encouragement and does not individualize instruction or interact positively with participants (Fox, Rejeski, & Gauvin, 2000).

Today, many exercise facilities are hiring individuals without the appropriate education. In some cases, people who call themselves certified personal trainers have no college education, no internship experience, and in fact, have only taken a written exam to become a "certified" personal trainer. Unfortunately, "certified" does not always mean "qualified." Ask yourself how someone with so little training can help a client who has arthritis, osteoporosis, a heart condition, low self-esteem, poor time management skills or a general lack of motivation to exercise. Some of the managers of exercise facilities who hire these people are only interested in gaining more memberships each year and care little about the people who are signed up and have stopped coming. When was the last time you received a call from the gym inquiring why you haven't been attending in a while?

Setting unrealistic goals—When beginning an exercise program, people sometimes set goals that are unrealistic and difficult, if not impossible to achieve (e.g., losing 10 lbs in the next week; turning fat into muscle; going from 0 days of exercise per week to 5). Many times, individuals look to change their entire life around to fit exercise in rather than learning how to fit exercise into their life the way it presently exists. Unfortunately, this does not work for very long. When the goals are not met, exercise is often stopped, thus forgoing all of the other important health benefits that might have been gained from exercise. In fact, after a short while you probably realized that this new change in schedule (e.g., getting up early to exercise; going to the gym right after work), while commendable in its intentions, simply does not fit into your lifestyle. So you miss a workout or two and before you know you are back to where you started-- not exercising at all. In order to have goals that work, you must set goals that are within your reach. They must be challenging, yet attainable. They must be measurable and modifiable, so that the focus of the workout centers on strategies and effort to reach these desired goals. Most important, they must excite you to get started exercising and motivate you to continue in the long-term. (In chapter 3, you will become SMAART and learn more about how to set goals that work for you).

Injury—A major cause of inactivity is injury. Clearly, exercise should be avoided when an injured body part is required for activity in order to allow time to heal. However, once the individual has been given a clean bill of health to begin exercising, that does not mean he/she is ready to start exercising again especially when the focus may be on the amount of fitness lost rather than being able to getting started again. Here's an example of how an injury temporarily stopped Steve from exercising and how he got back into his regular exercise routine.

Several years ago Steve, a regular exerciser since high school, needed to have surgery. He spent two weeks in the hospital and his doctor told him that he couldn't exercise for 8-10 weeks. After that period of recuperation, he got approval to start slowly, so he decided to go for a "little walk." Having always been used to running at least 3-5 miles, Steve thought the walk would be a breeze. Well, it wasn't. It took Steve 20 minutes to walk about a mile and when he finished his heart rate was sky high and he became depressed. Even though his physical injuries had healed, Steve was upset that his fitness level had dropped so low. Consequently, Steve considered stopping exercise altogether, but deep down he knew that exercise was the best thing for him and so he decided to continue and just start slowly combining walking with jogging and eventually running. For the first time in Steve's life, exercise was not a self-induced competition. Instead, it became fun. Rather than compare how fit he used to be prior to his injury, Steve was just happy to be exercising pain free. He began to set goals for himself to improve his present level of fitness (e.g., jogging 1-2 minutes longer each week; adding a day to his exercise routine). After six months of physical activity and exercise, Steve had now accomplished more that he ever could have imagined. Not only did he make significant improvements in his fitness, he was also enjoying and looking forward to exercising on a regular basis. (In Chapters' 6-8 you will learn how to develop health-related fitness programs that address you physical as well as your mental and emotional needs).

Lack of support from significant other—How would you feel if you began an exercise program, started to look and feel better, and nobody in your life noticed? Whether you choose to exercise alone or with a partner, it is so important to have support from a significant other, someone with whom you share the experience of exercise and the benefits that have been gained from being more physically active. When you don't get that support, it can decrease your level of motivation to exercise and makes you want to quit. In fact, research has consistently demonstrated that getting support from spouses, parents and significant others increased physical activity and exercise compliance rates for a variety of populations including mothers with young children (Miller, Trost, & Brown, 2002), cardiac rehabilitation patients (Erling & Oldridge, 1985) and children participating in competitive and recreational sports, structured exercise, and active leisure (USDHHS, 1996). Once you identify what support you need, you can then identify the people in your life that can provide you with this type of support (e.g., parents, spouses, friends, teachers) and thus enhance your overall exercise experience.

Boring—One of the drawbacks of exercise is that it can be boring. Whether it's sitting on the exercise bike for 30 minutes or doing the same exercises over and over again, exercise can seem a bit monotonous and boring. When you focus on how boring the exercise is, chances are you will lose the motivation to continue. However, there are many strategies that can be incorporated to not only decrease boredom, but to make exercise fun and exciting for you. Chapters 3 (goal setting) and 11 (cognitive strategies), are specifically designed to teach you how to have fun while exercising. I bet you can't wait!

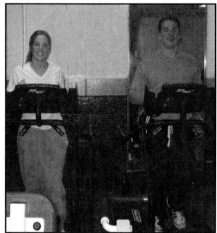

In conclusion, there are a variety of barriers that stop people from starting and or continuing to exercise on a life time basis. The first step in transforming exercise from something you should do and something you know you need to do to exercise being a significant part of your life is to identify the barriers that stop you. Now that you have done this it is on to Chapter 2 where you will identify your motives for getting started and hopefully continue exercising "now and forever."

REVIEW QUESTIONS

1. List at least five possible reasons for not exercising.

2. Which of the reasons you listed above have you used for not exercising?

3. Is finding time really a problem for you with exercising? If so, explain why?

4. Explain why exercise may be perceived as "NO FUN."

5. Why do you think some people do not get the results they want from exercising?

6. List two strategies that you can use to make your location to exercise more convenient.

7. If you were the owner of an exercise facility, what requirements would you have for your exercise leaders and why?

8. Explain why setting unrealistic exercise goals can decrease your desire to exercise on a regular basis.

LAB ASSIGNMENT 1.1

Are You Motivated To Exercise This Week?

1. How motivated are you to exercise this week?

   1   2   3   4   5   6   7   8   9
   not   highly
   motivated   motivated

2. Are you actually planning to exercise this week? If you answer "Yes" then move on to answer questions 3-6. If you answer "NO", then skip questions 3-6 and answer questions 7-13.

If "YES":

3. What exercises do you plan to do? _____

4. When do you plan to exercise? _____

5. Where do you plan to exercise? _____

6. For how long will you exercise? _____

If "NO":

7. Why have you decided that you will not exercise this week?

8. List all of the things that are stopping you from exercising this week.

9. List all of the reasons why you should not exercise this week.

10. List all of the reasons why you think you should exercise this week.

11. What can you do to motivate yourself to exercise at least one time this week?

12. Has your level of motivation to exercise increased? Please explain.

13. Do you still plan on not exercising this week?

At the end of the week, please answer the following:

14. For those who intended to exercise this week and did not, please answer the following:

    A. What really stopped you from exercising?

    B. What have you learned from this experience?

    C Do you plan on exercising next week?

D. If yes, list what you plan to do.

E. What are the chances that you follow your plan to exercise this week?

0%	10%	20%	30%	40%	50%	60%	70%	80%	90%	100%
No Chance										Very strong chance

F. What are the chances you will not exercise this week?

0%	10%	20%	30%	40%	50%	60%	70%	80%	90%	100%
No Chance										Very strong chance

G. List all of the possible barriers that might stop you from exercising next week.

H. Take a few minutes and think about possible solutions to overcome your exercise barriers.

I. How confident are you that you will incorporate the solutions to your barriers in the upcoming weeks?

1	2	3	4	5	6	7	8	9
not confident							extremely confident	

LAB ASSIGNMENT 1.2
(FOR EXERCISE SPECIALISTS MAJORS)

Applying Your Expertise

As a result of your background in exercise, you have been hired by a corporate exercise company to decrease the rate of exercise dropout in local exercise facilities.

1. Discuss five possible reasons why people drop out of exercise programs.

2. For each reason listed above, explain a strategy that can be incorporated to decrease exercise dropout and increase exercise compliance and adherence.

3. As an exercise specialist, describe at least three things that you would do to make sure you have met your client's needs?

REFERENCES AND RECOMMENDED READINGS

Bray, S.R., Gyurcsik, N.C., Culos-Ree, S.N., Dawson, K.A., & Martin, K.A. (2001). An exploratory investigation of the relationship between proxy efficacy, self-efficacy and exercise attendance. *Journal of Health Psychology, 6,* 425-434.

Cox, M.H. (1984). Fitness and life-style programs for business and industry: Problems in recruitment and retention. *Journal of Cardiac Rehabilitation, 4,* 136-142.

Erling, J., & Oldridge, N.B. (1985). Effect of a spousal-support program on compliance with cardiac rehabilitation. *Medicine and Science in Sport and Exercise, 17,* 284.

Emmons, R. A., & Diener, E. (1986). A goal-affect analysis of everyday situational choices. *Journal of Research in Personality,* 20, 309-326.

Fox, L.D., Rejeski, W.J., & Gauvin, L. (2000). Effects of leadership style and group dynamics on enjoyment of physical activity. *American Journal of Health Promotion, 14,* 277-283.

Franklin, B.A. (1988). Program factors that influence exercise adherence: Practical adherence skills for the clinical staff. In R.K. Dishman (Ed.), *Exercise adherence: Its impact on public* health (pp. 237-258). Champaign, IL: Human Kinetics.

Franklin, B.A. (1986). Clinical components of a successful adult fitness program. *American Journal of Health Promotion.* 1*(1), 6-13.*

Frierman, S. (2005). What's stopping us?: The role of higher education in increasing lifetime physical activity. Presented at the 2005 NAKPEHE conference, Tucson, AZ.

Genesis Personal fitness (2006): Your 1st step is to begin http://www.genesispersonal/fitness. com/CorporateFitness.htm

Gettman, L.R., Pollock, M.L., & Ward, A. (1983). Adherence to unsupervised exercise. *The Physician and Sportsmedicine,* 11 (10), 56-66.

Goodrick, G.K., Hartung, G.H., Warren, D.R., & Hoepfel, J.A. (1984). Helping adults to stay physically fit: Preventing relapse following aerobic exercise training. *Journal of Physical Education, Recreation, and Dance, 55,(2), 48-49*

Lox, C.L., Martin Ginis, K.L., & Petruzzello, S.P. (2006). *The psychology of exercise: Integrating theory into practice,* 2nd *edition , 10-11.* Holcomb Hathaway, Publishers, Inc.

Miller, Y.D., Trost, S.G., & Brown, W.J. (2002). Mediators of physical activity behavior change among women with young children. *American Journal of Preventative Medicine, 23 (2 Suppl),* 98-103

Shaw, S.M., Bonen, A., & McCabe, J.F. (1991). Do more constraints mean less leisure? Examining the relationship between constraints and participation. *Journal of Leisure Research, 23, 286-300.*

Teraslinna, P., Partanen, T., Koskela, A., & Oja, P. (1969). Characteristics affecting willingness of executives to participate in an activity program aimed at coronary heart disease prevention. *Journal of Sports Medicine and Physical Fitness*, 17, 224-229.

Thayer, R. E. (2001). *Calm energy: How people regulate mood with food and exercise.* New York: Oxford University Press

U.S. Department of Health and Human Services, (1996). *Physical activity and health: A report of the Surgeon General.* McLean, VA: International Medical Publishing.

Wankel, L. (1987). Enhancing motivation for involvement in voluntary exercise programs. in M.L. Maehr (Ed.),, *Advances in motivation and achievement: Enhancing motivation* (Vol. 5, 239-286). Greenwich, CT: JAI Press.

Weinberg, R. & Gould, D. (2005). Exercise behavior and adherence. *In Foundations of sport and exercise psychology (3rd edition,* 400-410. Human Kinetics: Champaign, Il.

Willis, J. & Campbell, L.F. (1992). Why people exercise: Motives for fitness. *In Exercise psychology pp. 3-7, 15-16.* Human Kinetics: Champaign, Il.

U.S. Department of Health and Human Services (2004). Healthy People 2010, Washington, D.C. U.S. Government Printing Office.

Chapter 2
Getting Started: What's My Motive?

In this chapter you will:

- Learn the variety of motives individuals have for exercising
- Determine what really motivates you to be more physically active
- Get prepared to exercise

WHAT'S YOUR MOTIVE?

If you are like most people, you start to exercise, then stop, then start and stop again. It's a vicious cycle. In chapter 1, you identified what stops you from exercising and being more physically active. In this chapter, you will examine the various motives individuals have for wanting to exercise. Once you understand what motivates you to exercise and be more physically active, you can structure your workouts to meet your motives and enjoy yourself while exercising.

In 1968, Gerald Kenyon developed a theoretical model that explained six motives people have for being more physically active (Kenyon, 1968a; Kenyon, 19868b). While other theories and models, like Health Belief Model and Social Cognitive Theory, have been more recently developed to explain what motivates people to be more physically active, it is Kenyon's work that serves as the foundation for much of what is presently used today both in theoretical development as well as practical application. Below are Kenyon's six categories of motives individuals have to be physical active and fit. Hopefully, one or more of these describes your motives for wanting to exercise. If so, then all you have to do is use exercise as the vehicle to help you satisfy these motives.

1. ***Physical Activity for Physical Fitness***—This motive focuses on being physically fit and improving the physical features of your body (e.g., toning your muscles; losing weight, etc).

2. ***Physical Activity/Exercise to Experience Vertigo***—Vertigo involves the participation of risky and dangerous activities usually derived from speed or acceleration. Activities in this category include sky diving, skiing, mountain climbing, snow boarding, kayaking,,

3. ***Physical Activity as a Social Experience***—This motive emphasizes the need to meet other people. Many people choose to exercise as a way of meeting with people with similar interests or enhancing the quality of already existing relationships. Consequently, exercise facilities often have classes designed to connect people of similar age, gender or interests (e.g., senior citizens; mothers-to-be), hoping to motivate people to rely on each other and to want to work out together (e.g., calling each other to set up a workout schedule; carpooling to the local exercise facility; signing up to take the same exercise class; encouraging and supporting each other;).

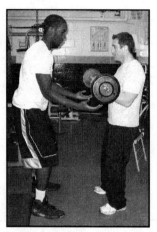

4. ***Physical Activity/Exercise as Catharsis***—An important benefit of regular exercise is its ability to relieve stress and tension in your life. Since exercise forces you to concentrate on factors unrelated to your stress and tension in life (e.g., how your body feels, your heart rate and breathing, muscular tension, form), you become distracted from your stressors, and replace those negative feelings with positive energy.

5. ***Physical Activity/Exercise as an Aesthetic Experience***—This motive relates to physical activity and exercise as a form of art and an opportunity for individuals to express their beauty, grace, and symmetry through structured movement patterns (e.g., aerobic dance, synchronized swimming, gymnastics, yoga, ballet, cardio kickboxing, martial arts).

6. ***Physical Activity/Exercise as an Ascetic Experience***—Exercise is viewed as a means to be challenged through intense, vigorous training in order to accomplish important personal goals (e.g., running a marathon, climbing a mountain, learning how to swim in deep water).

While Kenyon's motives have been and remain popular catalysts of individuals getting started exercising, research has discovered that there are several other motives that people seek to achieve through exercise. The first of these motives is for lifelong *health.* Specifically, as people get older, they sometimes realize they have not been living their lives in a healthy manner and thus have increased their risks for lifestyle illness and disease (e.g., heart disease, cancer, stroke, diabetes). Sometimes this ignites a wake-up call to start taking care of one's health by exercising.

Another motive to be physically active and exercise is for ***psychological well-being***. When people exercise, they often feel good about themselves for the efforts expended as well as the outcome achieved. In fact, research has found that exercise has been related to positive mood states with individuals expressing an increase in positive mood states (happiness, vigor, self-esteem) and a decrease in negative mood states (anxiety, tension, depression) as a result of participating in a variety of different physical activities (walking, jogging, aerobic dance, weightlifting, yoga, swimming). Consequently, exercise today is used as a means to treat and prevent people diagnosed with both acute and chronic mental and emotional disorders (depression, anxiety) and to improve positive mood states (vigor, happiness).

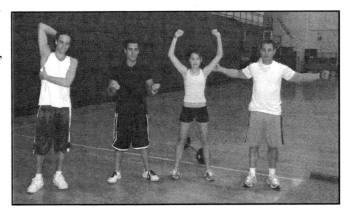

One final motive to exercise is *competition*. Many people thrive on competing vs. others and use exercise as a means to fulfill their need to compete by exercising with a partner and challenging each other to get to the next level, participating in exercising competitions (e.g., running events, dance contests), taking exercise classes and competing for maximum attendance, and hiring personal trainers to design exercise programs in order to achieve levels of fitness that have never been reached before.

So which one(s) of these motives work for you? Discovering what motivates you to want to exercise is an important first step in beginning an exercise program. It will help you to structure your program around your motives, thus increasing your exercise enjoyment and adherence in the long-term.

Now it is time to move on to Lab Assignment 2.1 which will help you to: (1) determine how motivated you are to start exercising this week; (2) identify any possible barriers that may stop you from exercising; and (3) help you to incorporate strategies to overcome these potential barriers. After that, it is on to Chapter 3, where you will learn how to set "SMAART" goals that are designed to increase your motivation and commitment to exercise as well as your performance.

REVIEW QUESTIONS

1. List Kenyon's six motives to be physically active and provide an example of each.

2. Explain what you can do to achieve each of Kenyon's motives by exercising.

3. How can you use exercise as a means to fulfill the motive to live a healthy lifestyle?

4. What psychological benefits can be derived from being physically active and exercise?

5. Explain the motive to exercise for competition.

LAB ASSIGNMENT 2.1

1. Circle the motive(s) that you interest you the most your to be physically active and exercise this week, over the next month and for the next year.

   Physical Fitness   Catharsis   Health

   Vertigo   Aesthetic Experience   Psychological Benefits

   Social Experience   Ascetic Experience   Competition

2. List and explain the actions you will take that will help you achieve your exercise motives.

3. Identify any barriers that may stop you from achieving your exercise motives this week, over the next month and for the next year.

4. What strategies can you use to overcome your exercise barriers this week, over the next month and for the next year?

After the week has been completed, answer the following questions:

5. Did you achieve your motive(s)?

         YES   NO

6. Explain why or why not.

7. How did it feel to exercise with a specific motive in mind?

8. Explain the actions you plan to take to fulfill your motives to exercise next week.

REFERENCES AND RECOMMENDED READINGS

Berger, B.G. (1996). Psychological benefits of an active lifestyle: What we know and what we need to know. *Quest, 48,* 330-353.

Beger, B.G. & Motl, R. (2001). Physical activity and quality of life. In R. Singer, H. Hausenblas, & C. Janelle, (Eds.), *Handbook of sport psychology*, (2nd edition., pp. 636-670). New York: Wiley.

Buckworth, J. & Dishman, R.K. (2002). Affect, mood, and emotion. In Exercise Psychology, pp 91-92, Human Kinetics, Champaign, IL

Dishman, R.K., Washburn, R.A., & Heath, G.W. (2004). *Physical activity epidemiology.* Champaign, IL, Human Kinetics.

Kenyon, G.S. (1968a). Conceptual model for characterizing physical activity. *Research Quarterly, 39*, 96-105.

Kenyon, G.S. (1988b). Six scales for assessing attitude toward physical activity. *Research Quarterly, 39*, 566-574.

National Heart, Lung, and Blood Institute. National Heart, Lung, and Blood Institute Report of the Task Force on Behavioral Research in Cardiovascular, Lung, and Blood Health and Disease. Bethesda, MD: Public Health Service, US Department of Health and Human Services; February, 1998

Statistics Canada (2005). *Physical activity by age group and sex* (CANSIM, Catalogue No. 82-221-X). Ottawa, ON: Statistics Canada. Retrieved from http://www40.statscanca/101/cst01/health46.htm?sdi=physical%20activity

Stephens, T., Jacobs, D.R., & White, C.C. (1985). A descriptive epidemiology of leisure-time activity. *Public Health Reports*, 100 (2), 147-158.

Teraslinna, P., Partanen, T., Koskela, A., & Oja, P. (1969). Characteristics affecting willingness of executives to participate in an activity program aimed at coronary heart disease prevention. *Journal of Sports Medicine and Physical Fitness*, 17, 224-229.

Thayer, R.E. (2001). *Calm energy: How people regulate mood with food and exercise.* New York: Oxford University Press.

U.S. Department of Health and Human Services (2000). Healthy people 2010: Volume II, 2nd ed. Retrieved from http://www.healthypeople.gov/Document/html/uih_4.htm$physactiv.

U.S. Department of Health and Human Services (2004). Healthy People 2010, Washington, D.C. U.S. Government Printing Office.

Wankel, L.M. (1988). Exercise adherence and leisure activity: Patterns of involvement and interventions to facilitate regular activity. In R. Dishman (Ed.), Exercise adherence: Its impact on public health (pp.369-396). Champaign, IL: Human Kinetics Books.

Weinberg, R. & Gould, D. (2007). Exercise and psychological well-being. In *Foundations of sport and exercise psychology,* 4th edition, pps. 398-413. Human Kinetics: Champaign, Il.

Weinberg, R., & Gould, D. (2007). Exercise behavior and adherence. In *Foundations of sport and Exercise psychology* (4th edition, 431-433 Human Kinetics: Champaign, IL.

Willis, J.D. & Campbell, L.F. (1992). Why people exercise: Motives for Fitness. In *Exercise Psychology*, pps. 4-17, Human Kinetics: Champaign, IlL

Chapter 3

Setting Goals: "Be SMAART"

In this chapter, you will:

- learn what SMAART goals are and how to use them in your exercise program
- create staircase goals that help increase your short-term and long-term motivation to achieve success
- identify barriers that stop you from reaching your goals
- develop strategies to overcome goal setting barriers in order to increase your exercise motivation and performance

When you decide to begin an exercise program, you usually have certain goals in mind. These goals can be the driving force towards increasing your motivation and commitment to exercise and improving your present level of fitness. It is important to note, however, that not all goals are equally effective. For example, if you set goals that are too easy and can be achieved without much effort (e.g., my goal is to exercise once per month) then you are not going to see any positive results and quite possible think that exercise is not working for you. Conversely, if you set goals that are too difficult or unrealistic, (e.g., run a marathon after a few weeks of training; develop washboard abs; increase exercise from one to five days per week; lose ten pounds in one week), you may become frustrated when your goals are not achieved right away and then lose your motivation to continue exercising in the long-term. Finally, if you set goals that are too vague, (e.g., I want to get better), the information you receive from your workouts may not be conclusive enough to determine whether or not you reached your goal. Thus, the problem is not so much getting people to set goals. It is getting them to set the right kind of goals-ones that provide direction and enhance motivation—and helping them to learn how to stick to and achieve their goals (Weinberg & Gould, 2006). This chapter introduces you to one of the most effective ways to establish and maintain high levels of motivation while exercising. Learn how to set goals that work for you rather than against you. The only criterion you need is to "Be SMAART."

SMAART GOALS

SMAART stands for: Specific, Measurable, Adjustable, Action-Oriented Realistic, and Time framed. Setting SMAART goals enables you to identify exactly what you want to accomplish, determine how close you are towards reaching your goal(s), decide whether or not you need to modify or change your goal, and identify exactly how long you think it will take to achieve your goal. Most important, the goals you set are completely within your control. Below are the definitions of each of the six components of the SMAART principle, along with examples of how to use SMAART goals. In Chapters 6-9, you will learn how to apply SMAART goals when designing your exercise programs for cardiorespiratory endurance, muscular fitness, flexibility, and eating healthy.

Specific—Specific goals are goals that state what you want to accomplish. Goals like losing weight, improving cardiorespiratory fitness (CRF) or getting stronger are all examples of specific goals because they state what you want to accomplish. Over the years, research has indicated that setting specific goals was more effective in increasing performance than setting no goals, vague goals or do-your-best-goals (Frierman, 1995; Gould, 2006; Hall, Weinberg, & Jackson, 1987; Weinberg, Bruya, Longino, & Jackson; Weinberg & Gould, 2003).

Measurable—In order for a goal to work, it must be measurable and put in numerical form. This way you know exactly how far along you are towards reaching what you want to accomplish. Although goals like getting fit and toning up specifically address why you decide to exercise, they are hard to measure since one day you may feel fit and toned and the very next day you may not. However, once you put your goal into numerical form, you can measure its effectiveness. For example, instead of saying that you want to tone up, set a goal for the number of abdominal reps you want to accomplish in today's workout (50) or the number of minutes you will run (25) without stopping. By setting measurable goals you will always be able to determine exactly how much you are progressing from one workout to the next. Most important, reaching these numerical goals will inevitably increase your motivation to continue exercising and make you feel better about yourself, too.

Adjustable—Setting a goal doesn't guarantee that you will reach it. For instance, if you set a goal to exercise three times in a week and you have taken the first five days off, you are not going to reach your goal. However, adjusting the goal (e.g., exercise one time in the next two days) allows you to stay on task and concentrate on accomplishing something worthwhile. Then when the week is over, you can focus on what you accomplished, exercising one time in the last two days, rather than on why you did not reach your original goal (taking six out of seven days off in the week).

Action-Oriented—To advance your goal(s) from actual words to accomplishment, you have to put it into action. In other words, once you set your goal, you should have a clear-cut plan of action that you will incorporate to help you reach your desired goal(s). For example, if you want to improve your muscular fitness, an action plan to help you reach you goal could be to go the gym three times per week and work two body parts per workout. If your goal is to eat healthier then your action plan could be to replace fried food with grilled or backed foods, eat fruit instead of candy, and drink water instead of soda. If your goal is to become more aerobically fit, your action plan could be to jog three times per week at a particular time (for example 5:00 to 5:30 PM) at your local gym or school exercise facility. By creating an action plan you take the goal from mere thoughts to actions.

Realistic—In order for a goal to work, it must be realistic and within your reach of accomplishing. The best way to set realistic goals is to first identify your present level of fitness and put that into numerical terms. For instance, how many minutes can you exercise continuously? How long do you hold a stretch for? How many sets and repetitions do you do in a muscular fitness workout? How many days do you exercise in a week? Then set a goal that is slightly higher than your present level of fitness that creates a reasonable and worthwhile challenge for you. For example, if you exercise 10 minutes without stopping, set a goal to do 11-12 minutes in your next workout. If you worked out two times this week, set a goal to go three times next week. If you held a stretch for five seconds, set a goal to hold for six or seven seconds. Finally, if you did six sets of muscular fitness work, set a goal to do seven to nine sets. Setting realistic goals allows you to be 100 percent in control of your progress.

Time Frame—Time frame is the amount of time you give yourself to reach your goal(s). In order for a goal to motivate you on a day-to-day basis, you must select a time frame that boxes you in and directs your energy and attention to get started right away and work hard towards reaching your goal. For example, if your goal is to start exercising four times per week, and you give yourself ten years to reach your goal, the chances that you are going to get started exercising right away are rather low. However, if you set a goal to exercise four times per week by the end of the month, you are immediately called into action. Each week you will have to decide the days and times that you will allocate for exercise. If you are progressing nicely (e.g., increasing frequency from two times to three times per week over the last two weeks), you will probably feel quite proud of yourself and have a high level of motivation to continue your quest towards reaching your goal of four times per week. However, if you are not progressing towards your goal (e.g., you went from three workouts in week two to two workouts in week three), you can immediately analyze what happened: Was it because you were lazy? Did you have a problem with time management? Once you find your answer, you can apply it to the next week and get right back into action (I will exercise on M, T, R, F from 4PM-5PM in the Recreation Center).

In addition to using SMAART goals, there are several other types of goals that you should consider when setting goals within an exercise program. Below is a list and description of the types of goals you can set that will help to keep your motivation and commitment to exercise high and your performance productive!

Set short-term and long-term goals—*Short-terms* goals are goals that can be achieved within a short period of time usually ranging from one day to one to two weeks. They are designed to keep you focused on what you want to accomplish right away (e.g., today's workout). Short-term goals provide immediate feedback that assists you in determining your level of progress. This regular progress check can help you to adjust your goals in the event that they become too easy or difficult. *Long-term goals* are more like dream goals. They define what you want to accomplish in the distant future and they provide the initial direction towards what you want to achieve, however, by, themselves they will not motivate you to exercise on a daily basis because they are too far in the future.

STAIRWAY TO SUCCESS

An effective way to understand the connection between short and long term-goals when starting an exercise program is to view them as a "***Stairway to Success***" (See Figure 3.1). The bottom of the stairs represents your baseline which is your present level of fitness and what you can do right now. The top of the stairs represents your long-term goal (what you want to accomplish in the distant future). Each step from the bottom up represents progress and the amount you are improving.

To get a clear picture of how to use the stairway to success, let's use the example of an individual (Archie) who has a long-term goal of running the marathon in 6 months and is presently running one mile without stopping. On the bottom of the stairs is the one mile that Archie can do right now (present level of fitness as of 1/15). The next step up is Archie's first short-term goal which is to be able to run two miles by 1/30. Each time Archie reaches his goal, he moves one step up the stairway until he inevitably finds himself closer to his one time long-term goal of running the marathon (top of the stairs) than to his original starting point of one mile. If at any time, Archie does not reach his short-term goal he can do the following: (1) give himself a little more time and set a new short-term target date; (2) put in another step in between the last goal he reached and the next goal he is striving to accomplish.

Set Positive Goals—Positive goals focus on what you want to achieve rather than what you are trying to avoid. By setting positive goals (e.g., I want to exercise three times this week) rather than negative goals (e.g., I don't want to take more than two days off in a row), you will feel better about yourself and what you are striving to accomplish.

Write Down Your Goals—Writing down your goals helps you to keep them in mind. Simply jot down what you want to accomplish on a piece of paper, index card or cell phone and place it in a visible area (e.g., refrigerator door, car seat, desk, day planner, computer/ screensaver) to remind you on a daily basis what you want to achieve. (See Appendix A: Weekly Goal Sheet.)

Have an Action Plan—An action plan consists of the strategies you develop to reach your goals. For example, if you want to exercise three times this week, your action plan should consist of the days and times that you plan on exercising as well as the place where you would like to exercise. This will help you to see how and where exercise fits into your daily life without having to make unrealistic changes. See Appendix B to use your action plan form to transform your goals from words into successful actions.

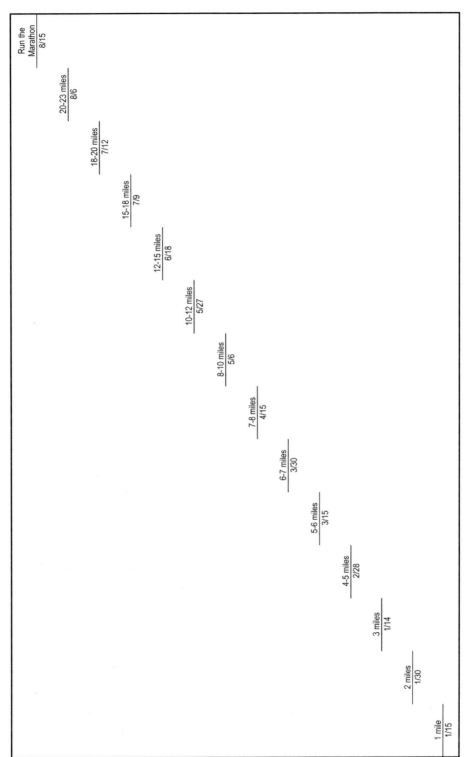

Figure 3.1—Archie's Stairway to Exercise Success

IDENTIFYING EXERCISE BARRIERS AND SOLUTIONS

Although goal setting can be a powerful motivational tool for exercising, simply setting a goal doesn't guarantee that you will reach it. Below is a list of five common barriers that can stop you from reaching your exercise goals along with possible solutions to minimize or prevent these barriers from occurring.

Setting Too Many Goals—The more goals you set, the harder they are to achieve because it becomes more difficult to track the progress of each goal set and determine what strategies are working or not working. For example, say that you want to improve your health-related fitness and you set weekly goals to go to the gym 5×, complete 100 minutes of aerobic activity (e.g., jog, bicycle, rowing machine), do 20 sets of muscular fitness training and stretch for 30 minutes. It is unlikely that you will be able to focus on all of these goals during your workouts because it is simply too much to concentrate on at once.

Solution: Set between one and two goals each week and that way you can stay focused on your goals and monitor your progress from one workout to the next, always knowing how much you need to do in order to reach your goal(s).

Setting Outcome Goals—Outcome goals are goals that are based on winning or doing better than someone else. The focus centers more on comparing your performance to someone else's than actually improving. Moreover, outcome goals take the emphasis off your own individual accomplishment and on to how well you are doing compared to others (e.g., my goal is to stay on the bike longer than the person next to me). Consequently, you lose control over reaching your goal because no matter how much you improve from your previous workouts, if your goal was to do better than someone else and you do not, then you don 't reach your goal and are left feeling frustrated and dissatisfied.

Solution: Set performance goals that focus on your own individual accomplishments. Compare your past performances (what you have just recently accomplished) with your future aspirations (what you want to accomplish in the immediate future—the next few workouts) and set your goals based on that.

Setting Unrealistic Goals—Unrealistic goals occur when you strive to achieve something that is out of your control and/or not within your immediate reach. This is common when you take time off from exercise and then try to start where you left off without realizing that you have lost some of your fitness and can't perform at the level that you used to.

Solution: Set goals that are based on your present level of fitness and not on what you used to be able to do or what other people you know can or strive to accomplish. Your goals should be just one "step" above what you can already do. This will increase your desire to work hard since your goal is completely within your reach.

Failing to Modify Your Goal(s)—If you consistently fail to reach your goal(s) week after week, you need to assess why you haven't reached your goals, otherwise you may begin to doubt your abilities to accomplish what you want and lose your motivation to exercise.

Solution: Modify your goal(s) so that they can be achieved. For example, if you set a goal to work on your flexibility for 20 minutes each of the last three weeks and the most you have accomplished has been five minutes then set a goal to do six minutes. In addition, incorporate a strategy for how you will increase your chances of reaching your goal (e.g., stretch before bed; stretch after lunch).

No Follow-Up and Evaluation—A big problem that many exercisers have is setting goals at the beginning of the week and then not using them in their workouts. As each day passes, the importance of the goals appears forgotten until the start of the new week when the individual realizes that he/she did not put his/her goals into action.

Solution: Develop a follow-up and evaluation plan and set up a time where you will examine it critically to determine the effectiveness of the goals you recently set. (Weinberg & Gould, 2003) This will help you to see if your goals motivated you to exercise, increased your performance, improved your self-efficacy and made exercise more fun for you.

In conclusion, goal setting is one of the most effective ways to increase motivation to exercise. Setting "SMAART goals" allows you to identify exact what it is that you want to accomplish and then provide you with strategies that increase your chances for success. Setting stairway to success goals enables you to visualize your long-term dream goals and establish a clear pathway of success by focusing on reaching your short-term goals, one step at a time. Identifying your barriers that may stop you from reaching your goals can help you to create strategies that can develop and sustain high levels of motivation and keep you committed to being physically active and fit for a lifetime. So, just remember when it comes time for you to set your exercise goals, write them down and BE SMAART!

REVIEW QUESTIONS

1. What are the drawbacks of setting goals that are too easy or too hard?

2. What does SMAART stand for? Provide a goal setting example for each of the six SMAART criteria.

3. Besides SMAART goals, list and describe several other goals that you can set while exercising.

4. Explain the purpose(s) of setting staircase goals.

5. Describe the benefits of setting positive over negative goals.

6. What are the purposes of having an action plan when setting exercise goals?

7. List three to five exercise barriers that can stop you from reaching your exercise goals.

8. What solutions do you have to minimize and/or prevent the exercise barriers you identified in question 7?

LAB ASSIGNMENT 3.1

1. List one to two SMAART goals that you would like to set over the next week and write them down in the space provided below.

   My exercise goal for this week is _____

   My exercise goal for this week is _____

2. For each goal listed above, develop your action plan for how you will reach your goal.

   Days of the week you plan to exercise _____

   Time of the day you plan to exercise _____

   Place where you plan to exercise _____

   What do you plan to do to reach your goal _____

3. Using your present level of fitness and recent exercise history (past 1-3 weeks), how realistic is/are the goal(s) that you have set for this week?

4. If you do not reach your goal(s) for this week, list the possible barriers that might stop you.

   A. _____

   B. _____

   C. _____

   D. _____

5. For each barrier listed above, create a solution that increases your chances of reaching your weekly exercise goals.

   A. _____

   B. _____

   C. _____

   D. _____

LAB ASSIGNMENT 3.2

1. Explain how you felt exercising with weekly goals in mind?

2. Were you successful in reaching your goal(s) for the week?

3. Did you enjoy exercising with goals?

1	2	3	4	5	6	7
not at all					very much so	

4. Discuss how your goals affected your enjoyment of exercise?

5. Did your goals affect your exercise performance?

1	2	3	4	5	6	7
not at all					very much so	

6. Discuss how your goals affected your exercise performance?

7. Are you planning to set exercise goals for next week? Please explain why or why not.

8. If you are planning to set goals for next week, you can use the weekly goal setting sheet in Appendix A and your Plan of Action Form In Appendix B.

LAB ASSIGNMENT 3.3

1. Using your "Stairway to Success" sheets located in Appendix C, select a long-term fitness goal that you would like to achieve over the next 10-20 weeks (Stairway 1) or 6 months (Stairway 2) and jot it down on the top of the stairway. Underneath your long-term goal, select the target date that you plan to reach your long-term goal by.

2. On the bottom step, write down your present level of fitness in numerical terminology and the actual date that you are starting to set your stairway goals.

3. Using the step just above the bottom, select your first short-term goal in numerical form and the date that you plan to be able to reach this goal by.

4. Each time you reach your short-term goal, continue to use the next step up the stairway to set your next short-term goal and target date.

5. If you do not reach your short-term goal on the target date listed, you should select another short-term target date 1-7 days later than the original date listed. If you reach your goal by then, you should continue to climb up the stairway by setting another

challenging short-term goal. Be sure to select a target date that is realistic to your present fitness accomplishments.

6. If you do not reach your goal by the second target date set, then you need to modify your goal by either adding a step in between your last goal reached and present goal not reached or crossing out the goal not reached and replacing it with a more realistic goal.

7. At the conclusion of the target date listed at the top of your stairway (10 weeks, 20 weeks, or six months, discuss the effects of using the stairway to success on the following:

   a. your motivation to exercise

   b. your level of confidence while exercising

   c. your level of enjoyment to exercise with stairway to success goals

   d. your level of effort and perseverance while exercising

   e. you're ability to identify and handle exercise barriers

   f. your overall performance using the stairway to success

   g. if you plan to use stairway to success goals again; explain why or why not;

   h. who would you recommend stairway to success goals for and why?

APPENDIX A—WEEKLY GOAL SHEET

Name _____   Date: _____

Below is a list of four categories that you can set your *weekly* goes in: (1) Cardiorespiratory Endurance; (2) Muscular Fitness; (3) Flexibility; and (4) Nutrition. Select 1-2 goals that represent the area(s) of fitness that you need to work on and are motivated to do so. Write down your goal(s) in the "Goal(s) Selected" column next to the category of goal that you have selected. Using the Seven-Day Chart below, record each day's workout next to the appropriate activity and under the actual day. After the week is up, add up your total workout performances and put them in the "Performance Results" column. If you achieved you weekly goal, mark an "A" across from your goal category in the "Achieved" column. If you did not reach your goal, mark an "NA" across from you goal category and under the "Not Achieved" column.

Category of Goals to Select From	Goal(s) Selected	Performance Results	Achieved = A	Not Achieved = NA
CRE Goals				
Frequency of Weekly Workouts				
Time in Minutes Exercised for Week				
Activity Selected				
Run/Walk				
Bicycle				
Elyptical				
Rowing				
Stairmaster				
Other				
Muscular Fitness Goals				
Frequency of Weekly Workouts				
Sets				
# of Exercises				
Increased Weight				
Flexibility Goals				
Frequency of Weekly Workouts				
Time in Minutes Exercised for Week				
# of Exercises Achieved				
Nutritional Goals for Week				
Fruits Consumed				
Vegetables Consumed				
Meals Planned				

	Day 1	Day 2	Day 3	Day 4	Day 5	Day 6	Day 7
CRE							
Run/Walk							
Bicycle							
Elyptical							
Rowing							
Stairmaster							
Other							
Muscular Fitness							
Sets							
Reps							
# of Exercises							
Increased Weight							
Flexibility							
Time							
Sets							
# of Exercises							
Nutrition							
Fruits Consumed							
Vegetables Consumed							
Meals Planned in Advance							

APPENDIX B—PLAN OF ACTION FORM

1. My goals for this week are:
   A. _____
   B. _____

2. In order to reach my goals, I will _____
   _____
   _____

3. I will exercise ___ times this week   1   2   3   4   5   6   7

4. I will exercise on the following days of the week: M   Tu   W   Th   F   Sat   Sun

5. For each of the day(s) I circled above, *I will exercise at the follow times and places*

DAYS	TIMES	PLACE
M		
T		
W		
R		
F		
Sa		
Su		

6. If I do not reach my goal(s) the barriers that will stop me are:
   a . _____
   b. _____
   c. _____

7. The strategies that I will use to stick to my goals and overcome my barriers are:
   a . _____
   b. _____
   c. _____

APPENDIX C FOR LAB ASSIGNMENT 3.3

Stairway to Exercise Success

Stairway to Success for 10-20 weeks

If you would like to use the Stairway to Success over the next 10 weeks, use the top step for your long-term goal which is 10 weeks from the time you start. Write your present level of fitness on the bottom step and set your first short-term goal on the next step above. Each step from bottom to top represents a short-term goal of approximately one week. If you would like to use the Stairway to Success over the next 20 weeks, each step from bottom to top represents approximately two weeks.

If you would like to use the Stairway to Success over the next six months, use the top step for your long-term goal which is six months from the time you start. Write your present level of fitness on the bottom step and set your first short-term goal on the next step above.

REFERENCES AND RECOMMENDED READINGS

Frierman, S. (2001). Be SMART: How to use goal to succeed in fitness. Presented at the Nassau Zone AAHPERD, Hofstra University March 15, 2001.

Frierman, S. (1996). Going for Your Goal: How to motivate your players in the off-season. *American Football Quarterly*, *2*, *1*, 64-65.

Frierman, S. (1996). The importance of setting realistic goals. *American Football Quarterly Mind Zone Section*, *2*, *3*.

Frierman, S. (1995). The effect of individual, group, and competitive goals on muscular endurance performance. *Journal of Sport and Exercise Psychology*, *17*, 51.

Frierman, S., Weinberg, R.S., & Jackson, A.J. (1990). The relationship between goal proximity and specificity in bowling: A field experiment. *The Sport Psychologist, 4*, 145-154

Gould, D. (2006).Goal setting for peak performance. In J.M. Williams, *Applied Sport Psychology: Personal Growth to Peak Performance,* 5th edition, McGraw-Hill.

Hall, H.K., Weinberg, R.S., & Jackson, A. (1987). Effects of goal specificity, goal difficulty, and information feedback on endurance performance,. *Journal of Sport and Psychology*, *9*, 43-54.

Kyllo, L.B., & Landers, D.M. (1995). Goal setting in sport and exercise: A research synthesis to resolve the controversy. *Journal of Sport and Exercise Psychology*, *17*, 117-137.

Locke, E.A., & Latham, G.P. (1985). The application of goal setting to sports. *Journal of Sport Psychology, 7,* 205-222.

Locke, E.A., & Latham, G.P. (1990). *A theory of goal setting and task performance.* Prentice Hall, Englewood Cliffs, NJ.

Locke, E.A., Shaw, K.N., Saari, L.M., & Latham, G.P. (1981). Goal setting and task performance. *Psychological Bulletin, 90,* 125-152.

Weinberg, R.S., Bruya, L., Longino,, J., & Jackson, A. (1988). Effective of goal proximity and specificity on endurance performance of primary-grade children. *Journal of Sport and Psychology, 10,* 81-91.

Weinberg, R.S. & Gould, D. (2003). *Foundations of Sport and Exercise Psychology,* 3rd edition, pp. 330-348. Human Kinetics.

Chapter 4

Principles of Health-Related Fitness

In this chapter you will:

- distinguish between health-related fitness vs. skill-related fitness
- learn and apply the eight principles of health-related fitness to meet your needs
- incorporate strategies to increase exercise compliance
- determine how to incorporate fun into your exercises

PHYSICAL FITNESS: HEALTH RELATED VS. SKILL-RELATED

Physical fitness is the ability of the body to function at optimal efficiency (Robbins, Powers, & Burgess, 2002). Someone who is physically fit is able to complete the daily demands of life and still have energy left over for leisure and recreational activities. In addition, someone who is physically fit can exercise for long periods of time at moderate to high intensities without getting overly fatigued (e.g., being able to jog for thirty minutes without stopping, performing 15-20 sets of resistance training exercises or stretching one's joints past

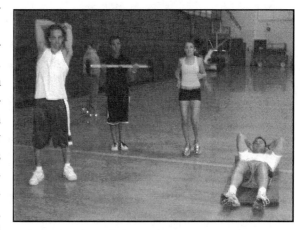

the normal range of motion without feeling tight or sore) (See Figure 4.1).

Physical fitness involves two components: health-related and skill-related. Health-related fitness concentrates on areas that are related to health (cardio-respiratory endurance, muscular strength and endurance, flexibility, and body composition) while skill related fitness emphasizes components that are necessary to succeed in sport yet are not directly related to health (agility, balance, coordination, power, reaction time and speed). For example, you can have a high level of hand-eye coordination and excel in sports like archery, billiards or bowling, yet not be fit in one or more components of health-related fitness (e.g., difficulty exercising continuously for more than a few minutes; unable to lift moderately heavy objects; poor range of motion in lower joints—hamstrings, quardriceps). Conversely, you may possess a high level of health-related fitness and be able to lift moderate to high levels of weight, perform aerobic exercises for long periods of time (e.g., 40 minutes) and demonstrate an excellent range of motion in your joints (e.g., you can touch your toes; vertically interlock your fingers behind your back, rotate your trunk all the way across your body) yet not be very athletic in sports.

In order to create a fitness program that addresses your health-related concerns and works for you (e.g., improving your cardiorespiratory endurance, increasing your muscular fitness, becoming more flexible, establishing the appropriate body weight), there are eight principles of fitness that you should first be aware of and then learn how to apply into your exercise program. Each principle serves as a guideline and addresses important information about the following: (1) what you have to do in order to improve your health-related fitness; (2) exactly how much exercise you should be doing in order to improve; (3) what exercises you should do in order to improve specific components of health-related fitness (e.g., cardiorespiratory endurance, muscular fitness, flexibility, body composition); (4) why you should focus on yourself and not others; (5) what happens if you stop exercising for prolonged periods of time; (6) how much rest you need after exercise overload; (7) the importance of warming up before starting to exercise and why and how to warm up properly; and (8) the importance of having fun while exercising.

In this section, you will be introduced to each of these eight principles of health-related and learn the value of incorporating them into your fitness program. Examples of compliance and noncompliance with each principle are included so that you get a clear picture of how to use each principle to meet your health-related fitness needs. In chapters' 6-8, you will learn how to apply each principle into your cardiovascular (chapter 6), muscular fitness (chapter 7) and flexibility (chapter 8) programs.

THE EIGHT PRINCIPLES OF HEALTH-RELATED FITNESS

1. *Principle of Overload*—in order to improve a system, you must place it under more than its usual amount of healthy stress. In other words, you have to do more than what your body is used to doing. For example, if you are living a sedentary lifestyle with little or no physical activity and you rode your bicycle for 20 minutes one day and took a 30-minute walk a few days later, both times increasing your heart rate from its' normal resting state, you would be doing more than what your cardiovascular system is used to and thus overloading that system. If you went to the gym and lifted weights that created some muscular tension that you weren't used to experiencing that would be an example of overloading your muscular fitness. Finally, if you hadn't stretched in a while (too long to remember) and you decided to stretch your major muscle groups (e.g., quadriceps, hamstrings, neck, chest, and back) by holding

each stretch at a position where you felt some tension for at least 10 seconds that would be an example of overloading your joints in order to improve your flexibility in those areas. In each example, you are creating a certain degree of work that your body is not used to causing what is referred to as exercise overload. By overloading your muscles your body begins to improve its functionality by getting stronger, improving resistance to fatigue, having more energy and feeling more flexible.

Compliance: Each week you do a little more than you did the previous week and increase any one or more of the following: (frequency-exercising more days per week; intensity-working harder; time-exercising longer). When you gradually increase your exercise load over a period of time, you begin to see improvements. For example, in Week 1 Linda exercised for 20 minutes per day on two separate days. In Week 2, she exercised for 23 minutes per day on two separate days and in Week 3, she exercised three times for 23 minutes each day. By increasing time per workout in week 2 and then frequency of workouts in week 3, Linda has succeeded in meeting the overload principle because she has accomplished more in each week than she was doing in the previous week. Consequently, her level of fitness is improving.

Noncompliance: Regardless of your intentions to exercise more, when you do less work from one week to the next (e.g., fewer minutes, fewer days per week, fewer reps) or if you take a few weeks off from exercising, you are not overloading. For example, last week Linda walked two times for 20 minutes each at a 15 minute per mile pace with her heart rate ranging between 60% - 65% of her max heart rate. This week, Linda walked one time for 17 minutes and her heart rate ranged from 40% - 45% of her max heart rate. As a result of Linda's decrease in frequency, time and intensity, she has not overloaded and thus her fitness level will not improve.

2. ***Principle of Progression***—in order to continuously improve, you must incorporate a systematic increase in the work that you do. Rather than deciding to do just a little more or work harder than your last workout, progression requires you to quantify exactly how much you plan to improve.

Compliance: You incorporate systematic increases into your workouts. For instance, four weeks ago, Melissa exercised two days per week and her workouts consisted of: (1) walking for 20 minutes; (2) performing 10 sets of muscular fitness training; (3) stretching for six minutes and (4) being able to reach her ankles when performing the modified hurdler's stretch. In order to comply with the Principle of Progression, each week Melissa set short-term goals to: (1) increase her walking time two to three minutes; (2) complete one more set of muscular fitness training than the previous week; (3) stretch for one more minute than the previous week, and (4) increase her exercise frequency from 2-4 times per week over the next 3 weeks.

As a result of reaching her goals, after four weeks, Melissa is able to walk for 30 minutes, complete 14 sets of muscular fitness training, stretch for 10 minutes and reach her toes when she does the modified hurdler's stretch. Most importantly, Melissa has now found the time to exercise four times per week.

By incorporating a systematic increase in your workout (e.g., adding a specified amount of time to your workouts, increasing the frequency), you are actually programming your improvement and thus guaranteeing success.

Noncompliance: You did not increase your workload (intensity, frequency, time) over the last few weeks. Perhaps you exercised one day instead of two, walked for 15 minutes instead of 20, and stretched for five minutes instead of six. Maybe you did absolutely nothing by not exercising at all. While it is certainly better to do something than nothing, in order to improve your present level of physical fitness, you must incorporate some form of progression into your workouts. The first step is to determine what stopped you from progressing. The next step is to decide what part of your exercise regimen you are going to increase from last week. Will you add a day to workout, increase an extra minute or two, add a few reps or select a new exercise to perform? Your answer to this question increases your chances of complying with the principle of progression and improving your present level of fitness.

3. ***Principle of Specificity***—in order to improve a particular area of fitness, you have to work that area properly. While this may sound easy, it is not uncommon for individuals to either select exercises that do not target the intended area of fitness (e.g., doing sit ups to decrease body fat; lifting weights to improve cardiovascular endurance) or selecting the right exercises yet work them improperly (e.g., lifting light weight in order to improve muscular strength; stretching to improve flexibility before warming up; jogging for five minutes to improve cardiorespiratory fitness).

Compliance: Mike has 32 percent body fat and he has decided that the best way for him to decrease body fat is to begin working on improving his cardiovascular endurance and eat healthier than he has in the past. He has selected brisk walking and the stationary bicycle as the exercises he will do continuously for at least 15-30 minutes two-three times per week and improve his cardiorespiratory endurance. In addition, Mike has decided to improve his nutritional habits and reduce his caloric intake by 200 calories by replacing two glasses of soda with water each day. By improving his cardiorespiratory endurance through walking and bicycling and decreasing his caloric intake by 200 calories per day, Mike has clearly satisfied the principle of specificity.

For those of you who want to improve your cardiorespiratory endurance, you should select activities that require oxygen and that you can do continuously for moderate (at least 15 minutes) to long periods (45 minutes or longer) of time (e.g., walking, jogging, bicycling, swimming, rollerblading) (see chapter 6). If your goal is to tone/define your muscles, then lifting weights that allow you to achieve 10-15 reps per set is an appropriate activity for you because you can select a series of exercises that will target each of the major muscle groups in the body (e.g., chest, back, shoulders, biceps, triceps, abdominals, legs) (see chapter 7). If your goal is to become more flexible, then you should work on stretching and familiarize yourself with the proper procedures for warming up before stretching and the various flexibility techniques to consider (e.g., static, passive static, PNF) (see chapter 8). Finally, if your goal is to lose weight (like Mike), you should combine cardiorespiratory exercise with healthy eating (see chapter 9). Each of these examples demonstrates how to identify the system that you want to work on and select exercises that are specifically designed to improve those components of health-related fitness.

Noncompliance: Mike's goal is to lose body fat and he chooses to lift heavy weights to strengthen his muscles and make his body look better. While lifting weights will improve Mike's muscular fitness, he will not lose weight this way since muscle weighs more than fat does. In fact, there is a chance that Mike may even get weight, especially if he is working out with heavy weight (at least 70% of his max) and eating poorly.

4. ***Individuality Principle***—everyone is different and progresses and develops at their own rate; therefore, the only comparison that is meaningful is between where you start and where you get to at some point in the future. Comparing yourself to someone else is meaningless and can be demoralizing.

Compliance: You focus on your own individual needs by first recognizing what your present fitness level is and then setting SMAART goals (Chapter 3) that will help you to improve at your own rate. You avoid trying to do what others are doing and instead set your attention on what is best for you. You determine how long, hard, and often you will exercise based on what your present health-related fitness needs and not what everyone else around you can or cannot do. Each new week, you can use your previous accomplishments to help you identify when and how much to increase. Doing so will inevitably create results that you will be proud of.

Noncompliance: You base your level of improvement on whether you are doing more or better than others. While many people have a natural competitive instinct, deciding how fit you are and how much exercise you should do based on what others do is not the most productive way to exercise because you can only control what you do (e.g., what exercises you do; how hard you exercise; how long you exercise; your present level of fitness) and not what anyone else does or how fit they are. Consequently, there is a good chance that you will feel dissatisfied and frustrated if you do not accomplish as much as your competitor, regardless of how much you actually do and thus reduce your effort to improve your health-related fitness.

5. ***Principle of Reversibility***—Wouldn't it be great if exercising was like a blue chip stock? You work out for a few weeks and then your fitness level improves more and more as the years go by, regardless of how little physically active you engage in. Unfortunately, you cannot bank your fitness. Exercising for a few weeks will not increase your fitness years later unless you follow the principles of health-related fit-

ness and continue to exercise on a regular basis. The principle of reversibility states that your body will adjust to the level of activity that it becomes used to. When you increase your level of physical activity or exercise, your body will begin to show improvements (e.g., you can exercise longer; stretch farther; lift more weights, improve body composition). However, when you decrease your level of physical activity or exercise, your body becomes de-conditioned and you will start to lose what you have gained. In other words, "if you don't use it, you lose it." In fact, the rate of loss will occur more rapidly than your rate of gain. However, not all levels of fitness reverse at the same rate. For example, cardiorespiratory and flexibility fitness reverse more quickly than muscular fitness. You can work as little as once per week on muscular fitness and still maintain your muscular strength and endurance. Conversely, you will have to work on your cardiorespiratory and flexibility more frequently (at least 3X per week). Otherwise your fitness gains will begin to reverse themselves. On the positive side, once you get back into exercising, you will regain what you lost more quickly than when you first started (provided you haven't taken too much time off).

Compliance: This is the one principle where compliance is not recommended since complying with the principle of reversibility means you are not physically active and losing what you have recently gained.

Noncompliance: To avoid losing what you have gained, stay active and plan your workouts in advance. Recognize possible barriers (Chapter 1) that may stop you from exercising regularly (every week), and continuously incorporate strategies to overcome these barriers. During times when it is more difficult to "find time" to exercise (e.g., final exam week, paper due dates, deadlines at the office, prior family obligations), plan ahead and jot down the available times that you do have to exercise. Decide where you will workout and focus on all the benefits you will receive from sticking with your exercise program (e.g., more energy, greater self-esteem, feeling proud of yourself, decrease in stress, guilt, frustration, and self-focused anger, living your life rather than your life living you).

You are in danger with losing what you have gained when your barriers to exercise are greater or more intense than your motives or reasons to exercise. When you start believing that you really "do not have time" or that exercising is "no longer convenient" for you, you have put the principle of reversibility into motion.

6. ***Principle of Recuperation***—the body needs time to recuperate after exercise overload and if you don't give your body enough rest, your chances of injury increase, you are more likely to feel sore, and you may become less motivated to exercise.

Compliance: Just as you plan on which days you will exercise, the principle of recuperation requires that you also plan your day(s) off. The lower your level of fitness, the more time your body may need to recuperate because it is not used to the overload from exercise. Once your fitness level improves and your body becomes used to the demands of exercise, you will recuperate more rapidly from exercise overload, and you can exercise for longer periods of time and more frequently per week if you choose to. Therefore, when first starting to exercise to improve your cardiorespiratory endurance, plan on working 2-3× per week taking off 1-2 days (but not more than 3) per week. When exercising to improve your muscular fitness, work each major muscle group one time per week. This will allow your body the necessary time it needs to repair itself and get you back stronger, more energetic and ready for your next weeks' workouts.

Noncompliance: After a long period of not exercising, Brian decided to work on CRE seven days per week. He felt that more was better, especially since he had exercised regularly several years ago and achieved a high level of fitness. After exercising four days in a row for the first time in months, Brian began to experience muscular soreness as well as fatigue and he noticed a decrease in his exercise performance from what he achieved on the very first day. Brian then realized that he was overdoing it and needed to give his body 1-2 days of rest so he could recuperate from all the work he had been doing from the previous four days.

7. ***Principle of Warm Up***—before exercising, you need to get your body and mind warmed up and ready for exercise overload. You can warm up your body by increaseing muscle temperature which will enhance elasticity and provide better blood flow to the working muscles. One of the most effective ways to accomplish this is to select the same or similar exercises that you plan to do in your workout only at a lower intensity. You can warm up your mind by training yourself how to think while exercising (e.g., listening to music, focusing on your breathing). In chapter 11, you will learn how to create cognitive strategies that will teach you how and what to think during cardiovascular, muscular fitness and flexibility exercises.

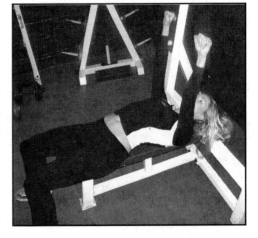

Compliance: The first step is to learn how to warm up properly. For example, before lifting heavy weights, determine the exercises that you plan on using for your workout and warm up with them by lifting weights that are lighter than those you plan to use in your workout (e.g., using 30%-40% of your max for about 8-12 reps on a bench press for a chest workout). If the lighter weights feel too heavy, you can warm up by using no weight and simply moving that particular muscle group in the same motion that you would during the weight training exercise (See Figure 4.2). Before participating in cardiorespiratory exercise, warm up by engaging in that same or a similar activity at a lower intensity (e.g., walking briskly before jogging; jogging before running; pedaling slowly before bicycling at your normal pace). Finally, before working on flexibility you should warm up your body by engaging in large muscular activity for a few minutes (e.g., walking or jogging on the treadmill before stretching your leg muscles). Warming up properly decreases your chances of injury and prepares your mind and body for exercise overload.

Noncompliance: Rather than walking briskly for the first five minutes, you immediately begin jogging or running at or near the speed you intend to maintain for the exercise duration. Rather than beginning a weight-lifting routine with light or no weights, you begin lifting weights that are at 70% of your max.

8. ***Principle of Fun***—in order adhere to an exercise program, you must enjoy your workouts and perceive it as something you like to do otherwise you will find reasons not to exercise.

Compliance: Identify what you perceive as fun and incorporate that into your exercise. For example, if you like to listen to music, invest in a small radio, I-Pod or CD player and use that while you exercise. If you like to socialize and/or meet people with similar interests, then find a partner with whom to exercise or register for an exercise class at your college or university, continuing education program, local exercise facility, or community center. If you like challenges, then try new exercises and set goals for yourself that take you to higher fitness levels that you want to attain. Consider entering competitions or races that challenge you to work hard (e.g., marathon, triathlon). Finally, if fun for you means being by yourself for a few minutes each day, then consider exercising alone and label that "My Own Quality Time."

Whatever it is that is fun for you, incorporate it into your workouts so that you look forward to exercising (See Table 4.1).

Noncompliance: You focus on factors related to the desired outcome of your workout (e.g., lose weight, tone muscles) rather than enjoying the actual process of exercising. Your thoughts are more on getting the workout over with than liking what you are doing.

In conclusion, the principles of health-related fitness are designed to guide in exercising properly and reaping all of the benefits associated with being physically fit. Learning how to overload and meet your own individual exercise needs, selecting exercises that address the areas of fitness you need to work on, making sure you incorporate the right amount of rest, being able to fit exercise in to your weekly schedule, warming up properly, and making your workouts fun are essential components in developing and implementing a sound exercise program that is certain to reward you with not only getting fit, but staying fit for life.

Table 4.1
Activities to Help Make Exercising Fun

Please check the appropriate box to determine your level of interest in selecting these activities while you exercise to make exercise more fun for you.

	Not Interested	Somewhat Interested	Very Interested	
Listening to Music				
Talking on the Phone				
Reading				
Playing Hand-held Video Games				
Watching Television				
Exercising with a partner				
Exercising Outdoors—Parks, Beach, Lakes				
Competition Races, Fitness Tournaments				
Community Events—Walkathon				
Other				

REVIEW QUESTIONS

1. Define physical fitness and explain the difference between someone who is physically fit vs. someone who is not.

2. List and define the components of health-related and skill-related fitness.

3. Give an example of how to exercise each of the components of health-related fitness.

4. List and explain the purpose(s) of the principles of health-related fitness.

5. Define the overload principle and give an example of how you can overload during cardiorespiratory, muscular fitness and flexibility exercise.

6. Define the progression principle and explain the similarities and differences between overload and progression.

7. Give an example of how you plan to incorporate the principle of progression into your cardiorespiratory, muscular fitness and/or flexibility workouts.

8. Define the specificity principle and explain how you can incorporate the specificity principle into improving your cardiorespiratory endurance, muscular fitness and/or flexibility workouts.

9. What is the individuality principle? What advice would you give someone who was upset that his/her friend was progressing more rapidly than he/she was?

10. Explain the principle of reversibility. What suggestions can you offer to minimize or prevent reversibility from occurring in your exercise program over the next six months to one year?

11. Define the principle of recuperation. Give an example of how you can incorporate this principle in your cardiorespiratory and/or muscular fitness exercise programs.

12. Explain the warm up principle. Give an example of how you would warm up prior to engaging in cardiorespiratory, muscular fitness, or flexibility exercises.

13. Define the principle of fun and explain why having fun is important to your exercise. Give an example of how you can make exercise fun.

LAB ASSIGNMENT 4.1

For the next week you are invited to begin exercising on your own. Select an exercise(s) that you are motivated to do over the next week and answer the following questions.

1. List the exercise(s) that you plan to working on over the next week.

   _____   _____

   _____   _____

2. Explain how you will incorporate the overload principle for each exercise(s) you listed above (e.g., exercising more frequently, longer, or more vigorously than you did last week).

3. How do you plan to incorporate the principle of progression into the exercises that you selected to perform this week?

4. In order to satisfy the principle of specificity, list the exercises that you plan to do for:
   CRE _____
   MF _____
   Flexibility _____

5. Explain how you are going to determine your own individual progress for each of the 3 components of health-related fitness mentioned above (CRE, MF, flexibility)..

6. Have you ever experienced the principle of reversibility? If so, explain how you felt about yourself and your own fitness level during this period. What strategies are you using to avoid the principle of reversibility?

7. Explain how your prescribed exercise plan for this week includes the principle of recuperation. In other words, how do you plan to rest each system?

8. For each exercise that you plan to do this week, describe how you will warm up before overloading.

9. What strategies do you have in mind to make your exercises fun this week?

REFERENCES AND SUGGESTED READINGS

ACSM Guidelines (2006). www.acsm.org

ACSM fitness book (2003). pp 9 3rd edition. Champaign IL: Human Kinetics.

Blair, S. (1995). Exercise prescription for health. *Quest*, 47, 338-353.

Blumenthal, J., Babyak, M., Moore, K., Craighead, W., Herman, S., Kharti, P., Waugh, R., Napolitano, M., Forman, L., Applebaum, M., Doraiswamy, M., & Krishman, R. (1999). Effects of exercise training on older patients with major depression. *Archives of Internal Medicine, 159,* 2349-2356.

Lox, C.L., Martin Ginis, K.A., & Petruzello, S.J. (2006). The Psychology of Exercise: Integrating Theory and Practice pp. 393-394. Holcomb Hathaway Publishers. Robbins, G., Powers, D., & Burgess, S. (2002). A wellness way of life. pp 50-110. McGraw-Hill.U.S. Surgeon General's Report. www.cdc.gov/needphp/sgr/adults.atm

Chapter 5

The Plan

In this chapter you will:

- answer seven important questions that will help you to develop your plan for exercising
- learn how to fit exercise into your life
- determine how to incorporate fun into your exercise

In chapter 2, you learned that people have a variety of motives for exercising (e.g., tone muscles, decrease stress, meet people with similar interests). When their motives are unfulfilled, they eventually decide there are other things that they would rather be doing and replace exercise with different activities (e.g., watching TV, playing video games, communicating with friends via e mail or cell phone; becoming attached to their i-pod). Imagine if you had a plan that helped you identify why you wanted to exercise, what you wanted to get from exercise, where you liked to exercise and how to incorporate fun into your exercise program. You would look forward to exercising more and probably find the time to get fit and stay fit, every week and every year for the rest of your life. This chapter invites you to ask yourself and eventually answer seven important questions that will help you establish a "Plan" for fitting exercise into your daily life. Several explanations are provided with each question so that you can begin to organize your thoughts and get back into action. The Plan start now!

SEVEN BASIC QUESTIONS TO GET STARTED EXERCISING

The Plan begins with these seven questions:

1. Why do you want to start exercising?
2. What do you want to get out of your exercise program?
3. With whom will you be exercising?
4. Where do you plan to exercise?
5. When will you start exercising? Time of day? Days of the week?
6. How many days per week will you exercise?
7. What do you like to do that is fun that can be done during exercise?

1. *Why do you want to start exercising?*

If you don't know why you want to start exercising, your chances of adhering to an exercise program in the long term are significantly reduced. That is why you should be clear about your choice to exercise. Is it because you want to lose weight and/or improve the way your body looks? Perhaps you want to get rid of the stress in your life or live healthy and reduce risk factors for lifestyle diseases. Maybe you want to meet new people with similar interests or perhaps your doctor has recommended that you start exercising. As long as you are clear as to why you want to start exercising, you can begin to view exercise as something that will meet your needs and give you exactly what you want. When you envision exercise as the vehicle to take you where you want to go, your motivation to find the time and get started exercising will increase. Once you have identified your motives (a.k.a reasons) to start exercising, the challenge becomes incorporating these motives into your exercise program so that you get what you want. Below are some common reasons why people want to start exercising along with strategies to structure an exercise program to match these needs.

A. *Lose weight*—This is one of the more popular reasons adults decide to exercise. As you get older your metabolism naturally slows down and if your level of physical activity has decreased and you eat poorly, there is a good chance you are going to gain some "fat weight." Simply put, you gain weight when you are consuming more calories than what you expend. Through exercise and eating properly (e.g., fruits, vegetables, whole grains), you expend more calories to help get rid of the unwanted fat. For more information on eating properly, see Chapter 9.

B. *Improve the way your body looks*—Exercise is a terrific way to shape your body and tone your muscles. In fact, there is no better way. As you will learn in the upcoming chapters, working on cardiorespiratory endurance (Chapter 6) will help get rid of unwanted fat and shape your lower body. Working on muscular fitness (Chapter 7) will help strengthen and tone your major muscles groups (e.g., chest, back, shoulders, legs, arms, abdominals) while also increasing body metabolism at rest. Finally, working on flexibility (Chapter 8) will help increase your range of motion and allow you to move freely and comfortably, prevent pain in your joints and lower back, and reduce the chances of soreness and injury.

C. *Reduce stress*—Everyone has some degree of stress in their lives. When things do not go your way (e.g., bad job; lack of finances; difficulty in school; overworking yourself; relationship problems, family spats), the end result is often negative stress "distress." However, experiencing stress is not really the problem. The problem is not knowing how to deal with your stress. One of the great things about exercise is that it can take your mind off of negative stress because it requires you to spend a certain amount of time thinking about what you are doing (e.g., correct form, pacing yourself, breathing correctly, reaching your exercising goals) and taking your mind off of your stressors (the things that create stress for you). For example, Leslie had just graduated from school and began a new job. Every morning she was required to meet with her boss and review her daily responsibilities (e.g., deadlines, expectations, work involved). Having grown up a perfectionist and always wanting to excel in everything she does, Leslie began to feel a great deal of stress in her life. Fortunately for her, Leslie became friendly with one of her new colleagues, Andy, who invited her to the local gym after work. He suggested that they go to the gym together three times per week right after work and take an aerobics dance class together. After a few weeks, Leslie's work stress had disappeared. She realized that going to the gym created a buffer to handle her work-related stress. Moreover, after work she felt invigorated and excited about her day and all that she had accomplished at work as well as in the gym.

So whether you are working on your cardiorespiratory endurance, muscular fitness, and/or flexibility, the exercises you do will require you to associate and focus on what you are doing for at least some period of time during your workout (e.g., heart rate, pace and time during CRE activity; proper form and breathing while lifting weights; tension point; length of time holding stretch for flexibility exercises). This will help you to take your mind off of your stressors and onto your exercise, thus decreasing your stress and making you feel better. In chapter 11, you will be introduced to cognitive strategies and learn how and when to program your thoughts while using associative and dissociative strategies. In chapter 12, you will learn more about the causes of your stress and how exercise can be used to transform negative stress (distress) into positive stress (eustress).

D. *Live healthy and reduce risk factors for lifestyle diseases*—In recent years, there has been a dramatic increase in the number of studies examining exercise for the treatment of lifestyle illnesses/diseases (e.g., heart disease, cancer, diabetes, hypertension, arthritis, chronic anxiety and depression (Lox, Martin Gillis, & Petruzzello, 2006). The results have generally demonstrated that exercise is an essential component in living healthy, reducing risks and treating individuals who have been stricken with these illness/diseases (Long, 1984; Long & Haney, 1988; Long & Stavel, 1995; Landers & Petruzzello, 1994; Blair, 1995; Blumenthal, et al., 1999). For those of you who want to live a healthy lifestyle, exercise is more than just an option. It's a necessity and a significant part of our everyday lives. By working on health-related fitness (cardiorespiratory endurance, muscular fitness, flexibility, body composition), you decrease the chances of acquiring these lifestyle illnesses/diseases and enhance the quality and longevity of your lives.

E. *Meet people with similar interests*—Many people join a gym or take an exercise class in order to meet others with similar interests. Although the desire to start exercising may have been with you for quite a while, the mere thought of doing it all by yourself (e.g., planning where and when to exercise, deciding what activities to participate in, having nobody you know around to communicate with) can be enough to deflate your interests to get started. However, once you find someone with similar needs and interests, you may notice that you are more motivated to start exercising. In fact, research has found that people who exercise in groups had a higher adherence rate than individual exercise alone (Dishman & Buckworth, 1996). According to Weinberg & Gould (2003), group programs offer enjoyment, social support, an increased sense of personal commitment to continue, and an opportunity to compare progress and fitness levels with others. Being part of a group also fills the need for affiliation as well as a greater commitment to exercise when others are counting on you. Today, many companies have corporate fitness centers or memberships at local exercise facilities designed to get their employees to exercise because they know that a healthy worker is a more productive worker. In addition, individuals often seek co-workers to exercise with so that they can get the necessary support and encouragement needed to stick with exercising. Finally, fitness clubs offer a variety of programs or classes in order to attract individuals with similar exercise and health-related interests (e.g., weight loss, body sculpting, spinning; yoga, cardio kickboxing). By focusing on similarities, people often develop a connection and look forward to spending time and coordinating schedules together which is a lot more motivating than getting yourself to go to the gym all by yourself.

F. *My doctor told me I had to*—Many people begin an exercise program because their doctor(s) had recommended it as a way to treat or prevent physical and mental illness (e.g., heart problems, obesity, arthritis, hypertension, cancer, anxiety, depression). While the doctor's recommendation is an important factor in getting these individuals started exercising in the short-term, it is usually not a sufficient source of motivation to keep them exercising in the long-term (over six months). In fact, research has demonstrated that the average dropout rate for cardiac patients was between 44% and 48% (Franklin, 1988; Erling & Olridge, 1985). Factors such as insurance running out, check-ups with the doctor decreasing over time, and a lack of knowledge of how to exercise properly by yourself have all contributed to the decline in exercise participation. In fact, the only way exercise tends to continue is if the individual finds something that he/she enjoys from exercising (e.g., an exercise partner, inviting facility, seeing results).

2. *What do you want to get out of the program?*

Now that you have made the decision to start exercising, it is time to identify what you want to get out of it. Whether your goal is losing weight or toning up, meeting people with similar interests or reducing stress in your life, increasing your self-esteem or mastering fitness-oriented challenges, you should identify what you would like to get out of exercising so that you can make the choices that work best for you and give you what you want. You can start by making a list of all the activities/exercises that you like and familiarize yourself with the benefits of each. Remember that the exercises you choose should work to improve one or more components of health-related fitness (cardiorespiratory endurance, muscular fitness, flexibility, appropriate body composition/eating healthy). In chapters 6-9, you will develop a more comprehensive understanding of each component of health-related fitness. Table 5.1 displays a list of activities/exercises that you can choose to help to accomplish what you want.

Table 5.1
Activities/Exercises That Can Help To Improve Health-Related Fitness

Activities/Exercises	Components of Health-Related Fitness Being Emphasized
Aerobic Dance	Cardiorespiratory Endurance, Muscular Fitness
Bicycling	Cardiorespiratory Endurance
Calisthenics	Cardiorespiratory Endurance
Cardio-kickboxing	Cardiorespiratory Endurance
Circuit Training	Cardiorespiratory Endurance, Muscular Fitness
Cross-country skiing	Cardiorespiratory Endurance
Heavyhands	Cardiorespiratory Endurance, Muscular Fitness
Hiking	Cardiorespiratory Endurance
Ice Skating	Cardiorespiratory Endurance
Jogging/Running	Cardiorespiratory Endurance
Jump Rope	Cardiorespiratory Endurance, Muscular Fitness
Roller Blading	Cardiorespiratory Endurance
Martial Arts	Muscular Fitness, Flexibility
Spinning	Cardiorespiratory Endurance
Stability Ball Training	Muscular Fitness, Flexibility
Stair Climbing	Cardiorespiratory Endurance
Swimming	Cardiorespiratory Endurance
Walking	Cardiorespiratory Endurance
Water Aerobics	Cardiorespiratory Endurance, Muscular Fitness
Weight Training	Muscular Fitness
Yoga	Flexibility, Muscular Fitness
Yokibics	Cardiorespiratory Endurance, Muscular Fitness, Flexibility

*Traditional sports (i.e., baseball, basketball, football, hockey, racquetball, soccer, softball, tennis, volleyball) were omitted because they address skill-related fitness more than health-related fitness on a recreational level. These activities can improve physical activity and to a lesser extent health-related fitness, if modified properly.

3. *With whom will you exercise?*

The people with whom you exercise with or without can play an important role in your overall enjoyment of exercise. Some people like to exercise alone. They view exercise as "their own quality time," and they want to focus on themselves, how their body feels and how well they are doing. Some individuals like to work out with a partner or in small groups because it provides an opportunity to socialize with people of similar interests, make new friends or simply to catch up with old friends. This can provide a distraction from exercise which can make the workout time go by more quickly. It can provide a source of motivation, encouragement and support that many people need in order to give just a little more effort than might seem possible if they were exercising by themselves. Finally, for some people, exercising with a partner creates an opportunity to get together with someone they may not be able to see otherwise. (e.g., incompatible schedules, live far away from each other, family obligations).

Whatever environment you prefer to exercise in, it is important that you structure it into your workouts. If you like to work out alone, then find a place that is empty or a time when your exercise facility is not crowded. If you like to work out with a partner, then look for someone with the same schedule and interests as yourself. Contact family, friends, co-workers or neighbors that you would like to spend more quality time with. Finally, if it is the

Table 5.2
Strengths & Limitations of Popular Exercise Environments

	Strengths	**Limitations**
Exercising at home	Convenient Comfortable Surroundings Inexpensive Private	Can be boring Lack of Equipment Lack of Space Distractions
Exercising at a local gym	Wealth of equipment to choose from State of the art equipment Variety of exercises to choose from Professionals to assist you Baby sitting facilities on premises	Membership can be costly Can get overcrowded Possible time limit on use of equipment Professionals may lack formal education in individualizing instruction to meet client's health-related fitness needs
Exercise in a college or university class	Expertise in instruction Opportunity to select from a wide range of classes Learn how to develop exercise programs that meet your needs Exercises are structured and scheduled for set days and times	Possibility of overcrowded classes Equipment may be outdated Facility may be old and run down Exercise time schedule is based on university schedule, not yours.

class or group scene that you're looking for, then contact a nearby exercise facility, community Y, or local college or university physical education or continuing education program to see about the courses offered in physical activity and exercise. For instance, many colleges and universities offer a wide variety of health-related fitness courses (e.g., aerobic dance, fitness for life, swim for fitness, weight training, yoga, cardio kickboxing, martial arts) specifically designed to address the health-related fitness needs and motives of their students. As their needs are identified and motives satisfied, students often recognize that they are not just taking the course(s) because they have to, but because they want to.

4. *Where do you plan to exercise?*

Whether it's at home, the local gym, community center, college or university, you need to decide where you want to exercise. Therefore, you should weigh the strengths and limitations of each possible site to see what motivates you to want to exercise in that particular environment. For example, exercising at home may be convenient, but it may also be boring and difficult, especially if you spend all day at home and you are around young children that require your constant attention. Exercising at a local gym can be rewarding if it is a well-run and well-equipped facility, but it may also be too costly for some people or unfulfilling for others if it is poorly managed and under-equipped. Table 5.2 provides a list of strengths and limitations for three popular exercise environments that can assist you in making the choices that work best for you.

5. *When will you exercise? Time of day? Days of the week?*

Sometimes even when you intend to exercise, you may run out of time by the end of the day and not get your workout in. Excuses like being too busy or not having enough time block your commitment to somehow get the workout in. The best way to ensure that you reach your exercise goal is to create a plan that includes the time of day that you would to exercise, the amount of time you will spend exercising, and what your workout goal is. It is important for you to view your exercise as a scheduled appointment, just as if it were a college class that you paid for, a doctor's appointment, sporting event or show that you had tickets for. You wouldn't think about canceling those appointments, unless you had an emergency, and that's exactly how you have to view your exercise: as a scheduled appointment. Write it down in your appointment book or day planner and treat your exercise time just as you would your other priorities, and stick to it because you're worth it!

6. *How many days per week will you exercise?*

National sources (ACSM, CDC, U.S. Surgeon General's Report) suggest that in order to achieve health-related fitness benefits individuals should exercise between 3-5 days per week. However, if you are unfit or just getting back into exercising after a long layoff, you may not be committed or ready to start off exercising this much. The good news is that you do not have to. As you learned earlier in chapter 4, as long as you are doing a little more than what you were used to (principles of overload and progression), then you will improve and achieve positive results. Therefore, be proud of any number of day(s) that you have committed towards exercising whether it be as few as one or as many as six because it represents an amazing starting point towards living a healthy lifestyle. Most important is the fact that you now have managed to find a way to fit exercise into your life without having to make significant changes. Think about it, isn't it easier to start out exercising 1-2 or 2-3 days per week and add a day after a few weeks than it is to go from 0 to 3 days when first starting out?

So, if you are a beginner or someone who has not exercised in several months or more you should start out slow (2-3 days per week at most). Remember that you cannot change your life around to fit exercise in. Instead, you must fit exercise into your life as it presently exists. Whether that is 1 day per week or 5 days per week, be proud and acknowledge yourself for making the right decision. As time goes by, you will be the one to decide if and when you are ready to increase days per week or minutes per workout. As you become more physically active and start to see results, there's a good chance that you will want to find more time to exercise. Who wouldn't want to put more into something that they were getting a lot more out of!

7.   *What do you like to do that is fun and can be done during exercise?*

Many of you may know how to exercise properly. You may know how high your heart rate should be during cardiorespiratory exercise, how much weight to lift in order to tone

Table 5.3
Activities to Help Make Exercising Fun

Please check the appropriate box to determine your level of interest in selecting these activities while you exercise.

	Not Interested	Somewhat Interested	Very Interested	
Listening to music				
Talking on the phone				
Reading				
Playing hand-held video games				
Watching television				
Exercising with a partner				
Exercising outdoors—parks, beach, lakes				
Competition races				
Community Events, walkathon				
Other				

your muscles and how long to hold a stretch for to achieve proper exercise overload. However, as mentioned in chapter 1, knowledge of how to exercise properly does not seem to be enough of a motivating factor to keep people exercising continuously for the rest of their lives. The fact is if you do not enjoy your workouts, you are not going to stick with it. Therefore, it is paramount for you to determine what it is that you enjoy and how you can make it part of your exercise program. So take a few minutes and jot down the things that you like to do. Then determine how you can incorporate these activities directly into your exercise program. Finally, take a look at Table 5.3 for a list of activities that you may not have jotted down that can be used to help you enjoy exercise.

So now that you have addressed seven important questions, it is time to really get started. Chapters 6-8 will help you to design your own exercise programs for cardiorespiratory endurance, muscular fitness, and flexibility. Each program will focus on your level of fitness (e.g., beginner-intermediate-advanced) as well as your level of commitment (e.g., low-moderate-high) to start exercising and live a healthy lifestyle. What more can you ask for? So let's get started!

REVIEW QUESTIONS

1. Discuss the benefits of developing your own plan to exercise.

2. Explain why people want to start or continue exercising?

3. What are some of the things that individuals like to get out of exercise?

4. Explain why some people like to exercise by themselves and others like to exercise with a partner or in small groups?

5. What strategies can you incorporate to help individuals exercise by themselves? in pairs? small groups? exercise classes?

6. Name three different places people can go to exercise. What are the strengths and limitations of each place?

7. Explain how planning the days of the week and times of the day can help someone to fit exercise into his/her life?

8. Why is having fun so important to exercising in the long-term (at least six months)?

9. What strategies can you implement to increase fun while exercising?

LAB ASSIGNMENT 5.1

1. Explain why you want to start exercising.

2. What would you like to get out of exercising in the next week, month, year and for the rest of your life?

3. Explain the benefits and limitations of exercising by yourself.

4. Explain the benefits and limitations of exercising with another person or in a class setting.

5. With whom to do plan to exercise with:

   by myself   with a partner   in a small group   in an exercise class   not sure

6. Where do you plan to exercise?

   at home   local gym   college or university   local Y/community center   other

7. Using the Exercise Time Chart, list the days of the week, times of the day and amount of time you will allocate to exercising over the next few weeks (Appendix A to use the Time Chart).

8. List the activities that you enjoy doing and can be done while exercising.

9. Explain how you will incorporate the activities you listed above into your exercise program.

APPENDIX A—EXERCISE TIME CHART

	MON	TUES	WED	THURS	FRI	SAT	SUN
6AM – 7AM							
7AM – 8AM							
8AM – 9AM							
9AM – 10AM							
10AM – 11AM							
11AM -12 PM							
12PM – 1PM							
1PM – 2 PM							
2PM – 3PM							
3PM – 4PM							
4PM – 5PM							
5PM – 6PM							
6PM – 7PM							
8PM – 9PM							
9PM – 10 PM							
10PM – 11PM							
11PM – 12AM							
12 AM – 2AM							
2 AM – 4 AM							
4 AM – 6AM							

REFERENCES AND SUGGESTED READINGS

ACSM Guidelines (2006). www.acsm.org

ACSM fitness book (2003). pp 9 3rd edition. Champaign IL: Human Kinetics.

Blair, S. (1995). Exercise prescription for health. *Quest*, 47, 338-353

Blumenthal, J., Babyak, M., Moore, K., Craighead, W., Herman, S., Kharti, P., Waugh, R., Napolitano, M., Forman, L., Applebaum, M., Doraiswamy, M., & Krishman, R. (1999). Effects of exercise training on older patients with major depression. *Archives of Internal Medicine, 159,* 2349-2356.

Dishman, R.K., & Buckworth, J. (1996). Increasing physical activity: A quantitative synthesis. *Medicine and Science in Sport and Exercise, 28,* 706-719.

Erling, J., & Oldridge, N.B. (1985). Effect of a spousal-support program on compliance with cardiac rehabilitation. *Medicine and Science in Sports and Exercise, 17,* 284.

Franklin, B.A. (1988). Program factors that influence exercise adherence; Practical adherence skills for the clinical staff. In R.K. Dishman (Ed.), *Exercise adherence: Its impact on public health* (pp. 237-258). Champaign, IL: Human Kinetics.

Landers, D.M., & Petruzzello, S.J. (1994). Physical activity, fitness, and anxiety. In C. Bouchard, R.J. Shepard, & T. Stevens (Eds.), *Physical activity, fitness, and health* (pp. 868-882). Champaign IL: Human Kinetics.

Long, B.C. (1984). Aerobic conditioning and stress inoculations: A comparison of stress management intervention. *Cognitive Therapy and Research, 8,* 517-542.

Long, B.C., & Haney, C.J. (1988). Coping strategies for working women: Aerobic exercise and relaxation interventions. *Behavior Therapy, 19,* 75-83.

Long, B.C., & Stavel, R.V. (1995). Effects of exercise training on anxiety: A meta-analysis. *Journal of Applied Sport Psychology, 7,*167-189.

Lox, C.L., Martin Ginis, K.A., & Petruzello, S.J. (2006). *The Psychology of Exercise: Integrating Theory and Practice* pp. 393-394. Holcomb Hathaway Publishers.

Robbins, G., Powers, D., & Burgess, S. (2002*). A wellness way of life.* pp 50-110. McGraw-Hill.U.S. Surgeon General's Report. www.cdc.gov/needphp/sgr/adults.atm

Weinberg, R.S. & Gould, D. (2003). *Foundations of sport and exercise psychology.* pp 414-415. Champaign, IL: Human Kinetics

Chapter 6

Developing an Exercise Prescription for Cardiorespiratory Fitness (CRF)

OBJECTIVES

After reading this chapter, you will be able to:

- Define cardiorespiratory endurance (CRE)
- Understand the benefits of CRE fitness
- Assess CRE
- Develop an exercise prescription for CRE that meets your needs
- Determine your level of commitment to CRE exercise
- Use SMAART goals to increase CR performance and motivation
- Incorporate principles of health-related fitness into your CRE exercise prescription
- Evaluate the success of your CRE program
- Learn how to prevent injuries while engaging in CRE activities

Did you know that the normal resting heart rate (RHR) is said to be approximately 70-72 beats per minute. With regular aerobic exercise this can drop 10 to 20 BPM or more. In fact, it is not uncommon for a resting heart rate (RHR) to be in the 60's, 50's or even 40's when you become aerobically fit. However, when you are aerobically unfit, your RHR can beat over 80 times per minute.

Imagine for a moment that when you were born, you were given a heart rate contract that stated your heart would beat 3 billion times and then stop forever. Having a RHR that beats 20 less times @ minute translates to 1200 less beats @ hour, 28,800 less beats @ day, 201,600 less beats @ week and over 10 million less beats @ year. (See Table 6.1 to determine how many times your heart beats in one minute to one year).

Table 6.1
How many times does your heart beat in one year?

RHR	1 Hour	1 Day	1 Week	1 Year
60	3600	86,400	604,800	31,536,000
70	4200	100,800	705,600	36,792,000
75	4500	108,000	756,000	39,420,000
80	4800	115,200	806,400	42,048,000
85	5100	122,400	856,800	44,676,000
90	5400	129,600	907,200	47,304,000

RHR indicates your resting heart rate or how many times your heart beats at rest

Wouldn't you feel better about yourself knowing that you chose to walk up a flight of stairs instead of having to take the elevator because you simply didn't have the energy to walk? Being aerobically fit will allow you to do just that and more. You will save millions of heart beats per year and not only will your heart beat less times per minute, but it will also give you more oxygen with each beat. More oxygen means more energy. Isn't it great to work so much less and get so much more out of it!

By now you should realize how important being aerobically fit is. Now it's time to develop the program that works best for you. This chapter will help you develop a program that meets your Cardiorespiratory (CR) needs as well as determine just how your committed you are towards becoming aerobically fit. Included are Exercise Prescriptions based on three levels of cardiorespiratory fitness (CRF) as well as three levels commitment. In addition, ACSM guidelines for aerobic fitness will be introduced and discussed in terms of both benefits as well as practicality. So have a heart and let's get ready commit to becoming cardiovascularly fit.

WHAT IS CARDIORESPIRATORY ENDURANCE (CRE)?

CRE is defined as the ability of the body to perform large-muscle activity at moderate to high levels of intensity for prolonged periods of time. CRE is an integral component of health-related fitness because so much of what we do requires the use of oxygen.

The Unfit Heart

Without a strong heart, a person may only be able to supply the oxygen necessary to perform minimal daily functions and thus be forced to reduce the amount of physical activity that can be done (e.g., walking up a flight of stairs, moving around continuously for more than a few minutes). An unfit heart has to work harder by pumping more often just to keep a person alive and thus, is subjected to more wear and tear than a well-conditioned heart. In situations that place strenuous demands on the heart such as running to class or catching the local bus or train to work, walking up several flights of stairs or carrying heavy packages to and from the car, the unfit heart may not be able to withstand the exertion. Consequently, the heart is forced to work harder by pumping more often, thus increasing one's susceptibility to heart disease.

The Fit Heart

The more fit a person's heart is, the more easily and efficient it works, thus providing more energy to be physically active without getting tired. When aerobically fit, the body is better able to consume, transport and use oxygen. With each heartbeat more blood is pumped throughout the body, blood volume increases, blood supply to the tissues improves, resting blood pressure decreases and resting heart rate slows down; the heart doesn't have to work as hard. Being aerobically fit further benefits the quality of life by helping to improve self-image, mood, cognitive functioning and the tolerance to withstand daily life stressors (e.g., academic pressures, difficult relationships with family and friends, uncertainly about job status, lack of purpose or direction in life, etc). Most important is the fact that as your CR fitness improves, you will reduce the risk of many lifestyle illnesses & diseases including heart disease, diabetes, colon cancer, stroke, hypertension, depression & anxiety.

BENEFITS OF CARDIORESPIRATORY ENDURANCE (CRE) TRAINING

By participating in Cardiorespiratory (CR) activities, you will be rewarded with a wealth of physical and psychological benefits that include:

Physical Benefits

1. *A stronger, more efficient heart*—Your heart will beat less times per minute and produce more blood to the working muscles. That is like having your car engine increasing in horsepower and giving you more miles to the gallon.
2. *Decreased risk of heart disease*—As a result of your heart becoming stronger and more efficient, your chances of heart disease have now decreased.
3. *Increased VO2 Max*—The amount of oxygen your body is able to use will increase. You will be able to exercise longer and more vigorously without getting as tired.
4. *Increased stroke volume*—Each time your heart beats, more blood is pumped. More blood means more energy.

5. ***Improved physical appearance***—As you increase your CRE, your body will begin to use more stored fat as a source of energy and help you get rid of some of that excess, unwanted fat. This is one time in your life that you feel better about losing than gaining.

6. ***Lower risk of lifestyle diseases***—By exercising cardiovascularly on a regular basis you will reduce the risks of many diseases associated with inactive and unhealthy lifestyles. These include heart disease, cancer, stroke, hypertension, and osteoporosis (just to name a few).

7. ***Improved immune function***—As you improve your CRE, you also improve your body's resistance to illness. As your fitness level improves, your rate of common sickness (colds, flu, etc.,) decreases.

8. ***Increased job productivity***—As a result of exercising, you will have more energy throughout the day to be more productive at work.

9. ***Better sleep***—As a result of exercise overload, your body will require more rest and this will help you fall asleep easier and improve the quality of your sleep, too.

10. ***Increase in longevity***—Being physically active reduces risk factors for premature illness and death which results in living longer. In fact, research has indicated that physically active people outlive their counterparts, as demonstrated by their lower overall mortality rate (Pate, et al., 1995; Blair, et al., 1998).

Psychological Benefits

1. ***Enhances appearance and improved self-image***—When you exercise you will develop better muscle tone, reduce excess body fat and look better. These changes will make you feel good about yourself, as yesterday's difficult workout becomes tomorrow's easy workout. The challenges you set and conquer will improve your self-esteem and make you feel proud of who you are and what you have accomplished.

2. ***Enhanced ability to handle stress***—By adapting to the positive stressors that exercise produces, your body becomes stronger and more resistant and better able to cope with some of the negative stressors associated with daily life (e.g., job, money, relationships).

3. ***Greater ability to relax***—After exercising, your body will begin to recuperate from your workout and your mind and body will feel relaxed, yet invigorated.

4. ***Improved mental functioning***—You will learn how to concentrate on relevant aspects of your selected activity (e.g., heart rate, pace, breathing pattern, etc). You will learn how to make effective choices within your workout such as knowing when to pick or slow down the pace, when you should go a few extra minutes and when you have had enough. You will learn what to concentrate on and when it is ok to dissociate and listen to music or carry on a conversation with an exercise partner. This will

carry over to other parts of your life as well and help you to be in control of your thoughts and think clearly and more productively.

5. *Help in preventing and coping with depression and anxiety*—Research has demonstrated that aerobic exercise has been associated with reducing both depression and anxiety with doctors prescribing a variety of exercises (including aerobics) as a way of treating each (Griest, et al., 1978; USDHHS, 1996; Morgan, 1997; Ryan, 1983). In chapter 12, you will have an opportunity to explore your own stress levels and learn exactly how your stress changes on days that you exercise compared to days that you do not.

6. *Enhanced quality of life*—One of the great things about exercise is that you begin to see your life more positively. The combination of both mental and physical achievements will help you to appreciate all that you have accomplished and all that you have to look forward to.

ASSESSING YOUR CRE

The purpose of assessing your CRE is to determine your actual level of CR fitness so that you can develop a program that will meet your needs and help you improve. Before participating in any of these assessments, you should practice them in order to familiarize yourself with their demands. Once you feel comfortable and confident that you can complete the test without overexerting yourself then you are ready to assess your CR fitness. There are several different assessments that you can perform in order to determine your CR fitness. Your selection of which CRE tests you can use should be based on the following criteria:

1. *Your current fitness level*—Each assessment has a different intensity or level of difficulty. The lower your CR fitness, the less intense the assessment should be.

2. *Degree of enjoyment*—Selecting an assessment that you like will increase your level of motivation and commitment to do your very best. If you select an assessment and do not like it, you may not try very hard and thus get an inaccurate assessment of your current CR fitness level.

3. *Facilities and equipment available*—Prior to beginning your CR fitness assessment, you have to decide where you are going to exercise and what equipment is available. Answering the following questions should help you to make the right decisions:

   a. Do you want to exercise at a public or private facility; in an individual or group setting?

   b. Is the equipment in satisfactory condition?

   c. How comfortable are you with using the equipment (e.g., track, treadmill, bicycle, pool, steps, elliptical, stairmaster, etc)?

FORMAL AND INFORMAL ASSESSMENTS

CR fitness assessments can be placed into two categories: (1) formal & (2) informal. *Formal Assessments* are more structured with a specific set of guidelines designed to create consistency in time, distance, pace, or rhythm. *Informal Assessments* are designed for individuals who possess a fitness level that is below the prescribed intensity, time or distance or are physically unable to withstand the over-all demands of a formal assessment. This section provides a description of some of the more popular formal and informal CR fitness assessments.

Formal CRE Assessments

1.5-Mile Run: This test is used to determine your CR fitness by seeing how long it takes to run 1.5 miles. This test is recommended for individuals who have at least a moderate level of CRE and can jog or run 1.5 miles continuously without having to stop and walk.

Procedure for the 1.5-Mile Run

1. Prior to beginning this test, you should make sure to warm up by walking briskly and then jogging for a few minutes followed by stretching (see Chapter 8 for a list of stretching exercises to consider).
2. Determine where you will run (standardized 440 yard track) or appropriately measured distance of 1.5 miles.

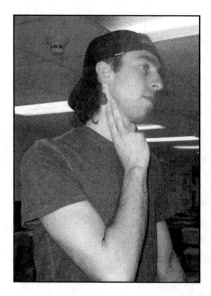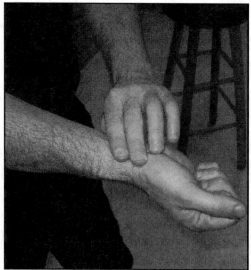

Figure 6-1—Assessing Your Pulse Using Carotid Artery and Radial Pulse Sites

3. If possible, bring a friend to time you and keep track of your lap times as this can help to pace yourself. If you cannot bring a friend then bring a stopwatch and calculate the time it takes you to complete 1.5 miles.

4. Pace yourself by running consistently. Use your stopwatch to compare times on previous laps and adjust future laps accordingly (e.g., slow down if you are starting to feel tired or get out of breath; speed up if you feel comfortable and have lots of energy left). Do not sprint as this will cause your heart rate to go up too high and create an inaccurate assessment of your true intensity for most of the run.

5. After completing the 1.5-mile run, record you pulse for 10 seconds and multiply by 6. This will tell you your heart rate. See Figure 6.1 to assess pulse using carotid artery and radial pulse sites. Then walk slowly for one minute and check your pulse again for 10 seconds and multiply by 6. This will tell you your heart rate recovery (HRR). See Table 6.2 for a conversion of 10-second heart rate to one-minute heart rate.

6. Cool down and continue to walk or jog slowly for another 3-5 minutes and then stretch your muscles in order to reduce soreness.

Table 6.2
Converting Your Heart Rate

10-Second Heart Rate	60-Second Heart Rate
15	90
16	96
17	102
18	108
19	114
20	120
21	126
22	132
23	138
24	144
25	150
26	156
27	162
28	168
29	174
30	180
31	186
32	192
33	198
34	204

Benefits of the 1.5 Mile Run are that it can be performed in a variety of locations (e.g., school yard, gymnasium, local fitness center, community park, close to home) and it requires a limited amount of equipment (running shoes, exercise clothing). *Limitations* include that not everyone is fit enough to withstand the demands of running 1.5 miles without having to stop. Therefore, it is recommended that before testing your CRE with a 1.5 run, practice a few times and make sure that you can run the entire distance without stopping. In addition, you should know how to pace yourself and be able to conserve your energy so that you can finish strong. Another limitation is that when the 1.5 run is used for testing large groups of

---

1.5 Mile Run Assessment Form for Individuals and Groups

Participant Jeremy

	Lap 1	Lap 2	Lap 3	Lap 4	Lap 5	Lap 6	HRAR	HRRL	RPE
Overall Time	2:10	4:20	6:25	8:25	10:20	12:10	28=168	21=126	16
Lap Time	130	130	125	120	115	110			

Here is an example of how to record your 1.5 run using a standardized ¼ mile track. In row 2, record your overall time each time you complete a lap. In row 3, calculate your individual lap times for each ¼ mile. This will help you determine your pace. Once you complete the 1.5 miles, take your heart rate for 10 seconds and record it in the HRAR (heart rate after run). Then walk for one minute and take your heart rate again and record it in the HRRL (heart rate recovery lap). In this example, Jeremy ran 1.5 miles in 12:10. He started out running his first lap in 2:10 (130 seconds). His HRAR was 28 beats in 10 seconds or 168 bpm. His HRAR was 21 beats in 10 seconds or 126 beats per minute. Finally, Jeremy indicated that his RPE was a 16 which indicates that he perceived his run to be hard.

Participant _____

	Lap 1	Lap 2	Lap 3	Lap 4	Lap 5	Lap 6	HRAR	HRRL	RPE
Overall Time									
Lap Time									

In the event that you decide to assess your CRE using a 1.5 mile run, this blank form is for you. Simply fill it out just like Jeremy did above. This form can be used in exercise classes, too. Classes are broken down into pairs with one student running first and the other student recording the overall and lap times, heart rate after run (HRAR), heart rate after walking for one minute (HRRL) and RPE.

Figure 6-2—1.5 Mile Run Assessment Form for Individuals and Groups

people in a class setting, individuals finish their runs at different times. If you are part of a large group, you can work with a partner and calculate each other's lap times, heart rates, RPE pacing, etc. (See Figure 6.2 to review the 1.5-Mile Run Assessment Form for Individuals and Groups).

12-Minute Run: This test is recommended for individuals who enjoy running for time rather than distance. It is also recommended for exercise instructors who test moderate to large groups of people simultaneously and may be pressed for time. Rather than measuring the time it takes to complete a certain distance as done with the one-mile walk and 1.5 mile runs, the 12-minute run measures the distance completed in 12 minutes. (Use Figure 6.3 to measure distance covered in the 12-minute run).

Procedures for the 12-Min Run

1. Prior to beginning this test, you should make sure to warm up by walking briskly and then jogging for a few minutes followed by stretching (see Chapter 8 for a list of stretching exercises).

2. It is best to use a standardized track or distance and measure off different distances around the track (e.g., 20 yards, 40 yards). This way you can determine the exact distance covered in 12 minutes.

3. Pace yourself by running consistently. Use a stopwatch to remind yourself how many minutes you have been running and how many minutes you have left. This will help you to determine whether to keep the same pace, slow down and conserve energy if you are getting tired or pick up the pace if you have lots of energy left.

4. After completing the 12-Minute Run, check your pulse for 10 seconds and multiply by 6

5. Then walk slowly for one minute and check your pulse again for 10 seconds and multiply by 6. Use Table 6.2 to convert your 10-second heart rate to a one-minute heart rate.

6. Cool down and continue to walk or jog slowly for another 3-5 minutes and then stretch your muscles in order to reduce soreness.

The benefits of the 12-Minute Run

(1) Many people can be tested within a short-period of time; (2) everyone is finished at the same time which is quite helpful for physical education teachers responsible for large numbers of students who are on a fixed time schedule. *The main limitation* is that some people may not be able to run 12 minutes continuously and thus have difficulty with the intensity of this assessment.

Name	Lap 1	Lap 2	Lap 3	Lap 4	Lap 5	Lap 6	Lap 7	Lap 8	Lap 9	Lap 10
	¼	¼	¼	¼	¼	¼	¼	¼	¼	¼
	½	½	½	½	½	½	½	½	½	½
	¾	¾	¾	¾	¾	¾	¾	¾	¾	¾

Circle each lap after completion. If you do not complete your final lap, you can record the fraction of the lap that you did complete. Each fraction represents a partial lap being completed.

Figure 6.3—12-Minute Run Assessment Form

12-Minute Swim Test: This test is similar to the 12-minute run test in that the goal is to cover as much distance as you can in 12 minutes while swimming instead of running. This test is recommended only for those individuals who are skilled swimmers and plan on swimming as part of their CR exercise routine.

Procedures for the 12-Minute Swim

1. Enroll a friend or swim instructor to time you for 12 minutes.
2. Make sure there is a lifeguard on duty and that he/she knows you are being tested.
3. Warm up by swimming or treading water for a few minutes and then stretching.
4. Pace yourself throughout your swim and swim as many laps as you can.
5. After completing your swim, use the RPE scale (see section on CRE exercise prescription intensity) to determine intensity (See Figure 6.4).
6. Cool down by swimming slowly or treading water for a few minutes.

The benefit of the 12-minute swim is that it is easier on the joints. **The limitation** is that not everyone is an efficient swimmer and while you may be cardiovascularly fit, you may not be an efficient swimmer and thus perform poorer than you would in other exercises that you are more efficient in.

The One-Mile Walk: This test is recommended for those individuals who are at a low level of CR fitness and/or unable to run because of injuries or pre-existing conditions that prevent running or other more strenuous activities.

Proper Walking Technique—Proper walking includes keeping your upper body upright (do not lean forward or backward), extending opposite arms forward (e.g., as you step with your left foot, your right hand should be out in front of your body).

The Borg RPE Scale

6	No exertion at all
7	Extremely light
8	
9	Very light
10	
11	Light
12	
13	Somewhat hard
14	
15	Hard
16	
17	Very Hard
18	
19	Extremely hard
20	Maximal exertion

Reference – Borg, G. (1998). Borg's perceived
exertion and pain scales.

Figure 6.4—Ratings of Perceived Exertion

Procedures for the One-Mile Walk Test

1. Select the site where you will walk your one mile. You can use a standardized 440-yard track and walk four laps or if you do not have access to a track, simply measure out a distance of one mile at a location that is convenient to you (e.g., around your block; campus area; office; local park).
2. Bring a stopwatch and measure the time it takes you to walk one mile.
3. Walk as fast as you can.
4. Once you have finished walking, immediately check your pulse by counting the number of beats in 10 seconds. (See Figure 6.1)
5. Multiply your 10-second total by 6 to determine your heart rate in beats per minute. Then walk slowly for one minute and check your pulse rate again for 10 seconds and multiply by 6.

The benefits of the One-Mile Walk are: (1) it is easy to administer; (2) it requires only a low level of CRE and (3) it is virtually painless on the lower joints. ***The limitation*** is that sometimes individuals may not know how to walk properly and think they are going as fast as possible, yet still not get their HR up enough to determine if they working at a sufficient intensity.

Step Test: This test takes only three minutes to complete. All you need is a bench or gymnasium bleacher 16 ¼ inches high, a stopwatch and a metronome (to determine pace). This test is not recommended for anyone who suffers from joint, knee or leg problems, is significantly overweight, or has problems with balance, coordination or walking up and down stairs.

Procedures for the Step Test

1. Use a gymnasium bleacher or a staircase that measures 16 ¼ inches high.
2. Step up-up-down-down to the beat of 24 steps/minute for a man and 22 steps/minute for a woman.
3. Practice going up-up-down-down for a minute in order to get into the proper rhythm and pace.
4. Perform the test for three minutes.
5. After completing the test take your heart rate for 10 seconds (see Figure 6.1).
6. Walk around for one minute and retake your heart rate.

The benefit of the step test is that it only takes three minutes to complete and it can be done with large numbers of people at one time in a variety of places (e.g., gymnasium, exercise facility, local park, at home). *The limitation* is that individuals may not be stepping to the correct rhythm (e.g., stepping more or less than the required number of steps) and have to adjust pace which may affect heart rate and cause an inaccurate assessment of the exercise intensity.

INFORMAL ASSESSMENTS

In case none of the CRE formal assessments listed above are right for you due to physical limitations (e.g., low CR fitness level, overcoming injuries, etc) or psychological barriers (lack of motivation, social physique anxiety—not wanting to be around others while exercising, etc), you should consider an informal assessment and follow the guidelines listed below:

1. Select any rhythmic activity that you like (e.g., walking, bicycling, jogging, elliptical machine, stairmaster, swimming, etc)
2. Record the length of time that you exercised continuously and the total distance completed (if applicable). For walking or jogging, you can also use a pedometer and record the number of steps taken. For the stairmaster, you can measure the number of floors climbed and for swimming you can count the number of laps swam.

3. Upon completion of your activity/exercise, you can check your heart rate to determine how hard you were working and use the RPE scale to evaluate perceived difficulty (See Figure 6.4).

4. You can use Table 6.3 to Informally Assess Your CRE and jot down your choice of activity, heart rate, post heart rate, RPE, minutes, distance, steps, laps, etc.

Although Informal Assessments may not determine your true cardiorespiratory fitness level due to the limitations listed above, it is your starting point and something to be proud of for the following reasons:

- you now know where to begin your CR fitness program;
- you have moved from a sedentary to an active lifestyle;
- you are ready to begin improving and set your SMAART goals
- your motivation to begin exercising should be high since you are not forcing yourself to do any more than you are physically or psychologically willing to do.

Table 6.3
Informally Assessing Your CRE

Use the table velow to record the activity that you select to perform your informal CR

Date	Activity	Minutes	Distance	Laps	Floors	HRAA	HRR	RPE

Assessment. Use the minutes' column to record the number of minutes you performed your activity before stopping. Use the distance column to record total distance achieved. You can use laps completed if you are assessing your CRE on a standardized surface (e.g., track, swimming pool with lap lanes) and plan to count how many laps you do. If you are using the stairmaster, you can record the number of floors climbed. Once you complete your CR assessment, immediately take your 10-second heart rate and record the total number of beats in the HRAA (Heart Rate After Activity) box. Then check your heart rate one minute later and record it in the HRR (Heart Rate Recovery) box. Finally, use the RPE box to record how hard you perceived your CR assessment to be.

Regardless of which assessment(s) you choose (formal or informal), your results represent your starting point towards improving and enjoying exercise. You now have valuable numerical information that will assist you in evaluating your CR fitness level (e.g., ran 1.5 miles in 14:00; heart rate was 160 bpm after completing the 3:00 step test; walked for 10 minutes and then stopped; climbed 22 floors in 12 minutes on the stairmaster). Most important, you can use your Stairway to Success (Figure 6.6 or review Chapter 3) to set goals to improve your CRE and get you ready for action. The important factor is not that you are less fit and unable to perform like you once did several years ago, but that you "got started" and for that you should be proud of yourself.

DEVELOPING YOUR EXERCISE PRESCRIPTION FOR CRE

Anyone who has taken prescribed medicine knows that on the bottle is information explaining what you are taking, the ingredients, how often and how long you should take it and what it is designed to do (e.g., fever reducer, cough suppressant, etc.) Well, like medicine, exercise has its own prescription commonly referred to as the FITT formula, which address the following four important questions about your exercise routine:

F—stands for frequency and addresses the question "How many days per week should I exercise?" It is generally recommended that in order to improve your CRE, you should do it three to five times per week.

I—stands for intensity and addresses the question, "How hard should my workout be?" There are two basic ways to measure intensity in your CRE program: (a) Heart Rate (HR) & (b) Ratings of Perceived Exertion (RPE).

(a) *Heart Rate*—an objective measure of intensity that uses your heart rate to determine how hard you are working; the higher your heart rate, the harder the workout is on you, physically. You should work between 50 percent and 85 percent of your heart rate reserve (HRR). (See below to determine how to get your HRR).

Lets use Sammy, a 20-year-old individual with a resting heart rate of 70 beats per minute (BPM), as an example of how to calculate proper intensity using HRR.

Predicted Max Heart Rate (pMHR) = 220 − age = 220 − 20 = 200

Resting Heart Rate (RHR) = 70

Heart Rate Reserve (HRR) = Max HR - RHR = 200 − 70 = 130

50%TI (Training Intensity) =	130 × .50 + RHR (70) = 135 beats per minute (BPM)
60%TI =	130 × .60 + RHR (70) = 148 BPM
65% TI =	130 × .65 + RHR (70) = 155 BPM
70% TI =	130 × .70 + RHR (70) = 161 BPM
75% TI =	130 × .75 + RHR (70) = 168 BPM
80% TI =	130 × .80 + RHR (70) = 174 BPM
85% TI =	130 × .85 + RHR (70) = 181 BPM

Using 50–85 percent of HRR, Sammy's proper cardiorespiratory (CR) intensity would be to exercise with a heart rate of 135 to 181 beats per minute. Individuals with low CR fitness levels should work between 50-70 percent and strive to conserve their energy so they can exercise for longer periods of time. As CR fitness improves, you will feel more comfortable

working at a higher intensity (70%-85%) while still exercising for sufficient time periods (at least 30 minutes). While using your HRR is the most effective way to maximize working at the proper exercise intensity, it can be a complicated procedure for individuals with no formal background in exercise. Therefore, a more simplified version of determining proper exercise intensity has been developed and implemented in both university and private exercise facilities. The formula looks like this:

1. Take your Max HR (220) and subtract your age.
2. Multiply by .50 to determine the low end of your training intensity and .85 to determine the high end of your training intensity.

For example, if you are 18 years old, then you would take 220-18 = 202. Then multiply 202 by .50 (low end) & .85 (high end). That would tell you to keep your heart rate between 101 and 172 beats per minute. This is also referred to as your target heart rate or area that you want your heart to be in while exercising in order to achieve maximal benefits. See Table 6.4 to determine proper heart rate using the simplified formula.

Table 6.4
Calculating Your Target Heart Rate "Simply"

Age	10-Second Rate Count	Target Heart Rate Range in BPM
17-20	20-29	120-173
21-25	19-28	117-169
26-30	19-27	114-165
31-35	18-27	111-161
36-40	18-26	108-156
41-45	17-25	105-152
46-50	17-25	102-148
51-55	16-24	99-144
56-60	16-23	96-139
61-65	15-22	93-132
66-70	15-22	90-131
71-75	14-21	87-126
75+	14-20	85-119

b. ***Ratings of Perceived Exertion*** (RPE)—Developed by Borg in 1971, the RPE is a subjective measure of exercise intensity that asks you to determine how hard you perceive your workout to be. In theory, the higher your heart rate is, the harder you should perceive your workout to be. However, some people like to exercise at higher intensities and they perceive it to be quite comfortable. Others, however, are not used to the sudden demands that exercise places on their bodies and may perceive a workout to be quite hard even though their heart rate is well within or even below their target heart rate. In addition, not everyone likes to check their heart rate during or after aerobic exercise. Having the RPE allows you to evaluate just how hard you perceive you are working and thus determine if you should increase, decrease or maintain the same intensity. To get a complete understanding of the Borg scale, you can read Borg's Perceived Exertion and Pain Scales (1998).

I recommend that you use both measures (HR & RPE) for the following reasons:

1. Checking your heart rate will provide you with the information you need to clearly see how hard your CR system is working.

2. The RPE scale will give you an opportunity to investigate you thoughts/perceptions about how you feel about the exercise intensity you are creating.

Using both measures maximizes working at the right intensity, thus making your CR workout challenging and productive rather than boring or painful.

T—stands for time and addresses the question, "How long should my workout be?"

Generally, it is recommended that you should exercise for 20-60 minutes. Of Frequency, Intensity and Time, Time is the most important component, especially for beginners or individuals with low level of CR fitness. By increasing minutes from one week to the next you are overloading your CR system and thus improving. In addition, increasing time is more practical than either Frequency or Intensity for the following reasons:

1. if you feel pressed for time, you are not going to be able to find more days in the week to exercise;

2. if you are just getting started exercising, increasing intensity too much may cause you to overdo it and become excessively sore which will not only decrease the probability you can exercise productivity in the next day or two, but it will also decrease your motivation to want to;

3. the hardest part of beginning your workouts is usually getting to the exercise facility; once you are there, adding a few extra minutes to your workout, not only increases your performance, but it will also make you feel good about yourself and increase your desire to do it again in the near future. So remember, it's **Time That Is On Your Side!**

T—stands for type and addresses the question, "What activities should I do? Any large muscle activity that is rhythmic in nature that you can do continuously for at least 15 minutes matches the criteria for the right exercise to improve your CRE. See Table 6.5 for a list of activities to choose from.

Table 6.5
CRE Activities to Choose From or Selecting Your CRE Activities

Aerobics (low impact) (moderate impact) (high impact)	Roller Skating
Bicycling	Rowing
Cardio Kickboxing	Running
Elyptical Machine	Skateboarding
Hiking	Skiing
Ice Skating	Spinning
Jogging	Swimming
Jump Roping	Stair Climbing (Stairmaster)
Kyacking	Tae Bo
Roller Blading	Walking

The most common way to develop a CR exercise prescription is to use the results from your CR fitness assessment and match your level of CR fitness to one of the three CR fitness prescriptions listed below. Choose whatever activities you like that will motivate you to want to exercise. There is no one exercise that you must do in order to improve your CR fitness. As long as you are working within your target heart rate between 50% and 85% of your predicted max heart rate, you will be overloading your CRE and improving to a higher level of CR fitness. See Table 6.6 to select an exercise prescription based on your CRF level.

Table 6.6
Exercise Prescription Based on CR Level of Fitness

Low Level of CRF

	WEEK 1	WEEK 2	WEEK 3	WEEK 4
F	3	3	3-4	3-4
I-HRR RPE	50-60% 10-12 RPE	50-65% 10-14 RPE	60-70% 12-16 RPE	60-80% 12-17 RPE
T	20-25 min	25-30 min	25-30 min	30-35 min
T use Table 6.5				

Moderate Level of CRF

	WEEK 1	WEEK 2	WEEK 3	WEEK 4
F	3	3-4	3-5	3-5
I-HRR RPE	60-70% 11-13 RPE	60-75% 12-15 RPE	60-80% 13-16 RPE	60-85% 13-17 RPE
T	25-30 min	30-35 min	35-40 min	40-45 min
T use Table 6.5				

High Level of CRF

	WEEK 1	WEEK 2	WEEK 3	WEEK 4
F	3	3-4	3-5	3-5
I-HRR RPE	60-85% 12-15 RPE	65-85% 13-16 RPE	65-85% 13-17 RPE	70-85% 13-18 RPE
T	40-45 min	45-50 min	50-55 min	55-60 min
T use Table 6.5				

DETERMINING YOUR LEVEL OF COMMITMENT

Over the years, scientific sources have suggested that you should exercise 3-5X per week for 20-60 minutes per workout (ACSM, 2005; Fahey, Insel, & Roth, 2005). While this recommendation may work for some individuals, it may not work for others. The simple fact is that if you are not committed to exercise then you will not do it for very long! How else can you explain the fact that only 15-20% of our adult population exercises enough to achieve health-related fitness benefits? As long as you continue to perceive yourself to "have to," rather than "want to" exercise then it is unlikely that you will comply with this recommended prescription for the long haul "the rest of your life." You may give exercise a try for a short while, but after only a few months, you will find yourself in the category of exercise "drop-out," along with the other 50-60% of the population. The bottom line is that you simply cannot change your life around to make exercise fit. You have to learn how to fit exercise in to your already existing life. This starts with identifying your level of commitment to exercise. In other words, what activities are you committed to? How many days per week and how many minutes per workout are you committed to? Your answers to these questions will help determine exactly what you will and will not do.

Three Levels of Commitment

A low level of commitment is characterized by someone who's motives not to exercise exceed his/her motives to exercise. Generally, these individuals are either not exercising at all or doing so at a minimal level because they feel they "have to" not because they "want to" (e.g., doctor's recommendation, have to lose weight). Frequency of exercise is inconsistent at best and as time goes by the mere thought of exercise is often replaced with the barriers that stop one from actually getting started.

A moderate level of commitment is characterized by someone who either wants to start or is actually exercising, but is concerned he/she may not continue. Although there is a genuine concern to get started and be physically active, there is some doubt that compliance (short-term exercise participation) and ultimately adherence (long-term exercise participation) will occur. Attempts are made to exercise and sometimes achieved, however, consistency is lacking and exercise benefits are achieved sporadically.

A high level of commitment is characterized by someone who is able to fit exercise into his/her life. This individual looks forward to exercise, has positive thoughts about doing it, and feels great afterward. Uncertainty of where and when to exercise or of how to enjoy and be motivated to exercise have clearly been replaced with feelings of pride and accomplishment, confidence and self-desire to exercise.

So where are you on the commitment scale?

| 1 | 2 | 3 | 4 | 5 | 6 | 7 | 8 | 9 |

Low commitment   **Moderate Commitment**   **High Commitment**

How many days per week and minutes per workout will you commit to exercise? Once you know exactly what you are committed to, you will miraculously find the time to exercise. You will feel good about what you are accomplishing and as time goes by, you will suddenly find more time to exercise because you "choose to" rather than because you "have to." Based upon your level of commitment, you should consider one of the three four-week cardiorespiratory fitness (CRF) programs listed in Table 6.7. Select the program that you have the highest commitment level to participate in. In other words, do what you want to do, not what you think you should do.

Table 6.7
CR Exercise Frequency Based on Level of Commitment

	Week 1	Week 2	Week 3	Week 4
Low	1-2	1-2	2	2-3
Moderate	2-3	3	3-4	3-4
High	3-5	3-5	4-5	4-6

USING SMAART GOALS TO INCREASE CR FITNESS AND MOTIVATION

In chapter 3, you were introduced to goal setting and learned the value of setting SMAART goals. Now it is time to incorporate SMAART goals into your CR fitness program so that you can increase your exercise performance as well as create or maintain a high level of exercise motivation. To illustrate how to use SMAART goals with your CR fitness program, let's use Arline as an example.

Presently, Arline is able to perform 15 minutes of CR activity, including jogging for 11 minutes and then biking for four minutes on level 1. Using the SMAART principle, Arline sets the following goals.

Goals	Arline's SMAART Goals	Your SMAART Goals
SPECIFIC	Improve CRF	
MEASURABLE	Be able to jog & bike continuously for 20 minutes	
ACTION-ORIENTED	Run and bike 2-3× per week starting at 15-16 minutes in week 1; 16-18 minutes in week 2 & 18-20 minutes in week 3	
ADJUSTABLE	If the action is not achieved in week 1, Arline will either decrease 1-2 minutes or include walking into her actions	
REALISTIC	Arline has set her goal based on his present level of CR fitness	
TIME-FRAME	Arline would like to reach her goal within 3 weeks.	

Figure 6.5—Using SMAART Goals to Increase CRF and Motivation Goals

As you can see, Arline has a plan to improve her CRF by modestly increasing her workouts from 16 to 20 minutes over a three-week period. In addition, Arline has a backup plan to adjust her goal, in the event that she does not reach her desired performance. Finally, Arline has selected several different activities to choose from to help her reach her goals. By setting SMAART goals Arline has increased her chances of improving her CR fitness and as she begins to see progress from weeks 1 to week 3, Arline should experience an increase in her motivation to continue working on his CR fitness, too.

In addition to setting SMAART goals, if you have CR fitness goals that you think may take longer than a few weeks to achieve, you can use Stairway to Success (STS) goals presented in Chapter 3. Here are two examples of how to use STS goals to improve your CRE.

First, lets use Marc, a college student who used to run in high school but since has taken several years off and decided it was time to improve his CRE once and for all so he enrolled in Fitness for Life and ran 1.5 miles in 16:00 on 1/15. Using the STS, Marc has established both short-term and long-term goals along with target dates for reaching his goals. His long-term goal by 7/31 is to run 1.5 miles in under 12:00. In order to get there Marc will need to focus on his short-term goals and take one step at a time. His first short-term goal in two weeks (1/31) is to run 1.5 miles in 15:50. After Marc reaches that goal, he will move up to the next step where his goal is 15:25 by 2/14. As you can see, each step up from Marc's baseline is specific, measurable, realistic and challenging. Moreover, as Marc progresses from one step to the next, hew gets closer to reaching his long-term goal of running 1.5 miles in 12:00 which should certainly help him to increase his confidence, motivation and commitment to continue improving.

Now lets move onto Mae, a middle-aged family-oriented career woman who wants to increase her CRE by walking longer amounts of time. Her ideal, long-term dream goal is to be able to walk continuously for 40 minutes by 7/31. Presently, she is able to walk for 10 minutes without stopping. Every two weeks Mae has set her short-term goals to increasing walking by 2-3 minutes. Each time she reaches her short-term goal, Mae will move one step up and progress closer and closer to her long-term goal and thus increase her confidence, motivation, and commitment to be cardiovascularly fit (just like Marc). See Figure 6.6 to review how Marc and Mae climbed the STS to reach their goals. Let's take full advantage and learn from Marc and Mae. Use the Stairway to improve your CRE, too.

At the conclusion of this chapter, you will be able to set your own goals using both SMAART and Staircase formats to guide you to improving your CRF and increasing your motivation to stay fit. You are also invited to review chapter 3 and use the weekly goal sheets (in a SMAART way of course). A copy of the weekly goal and the stairway to success goal sheets are included in Appendix 6A and Appendix 6B for you to use for your CRE program.

APPLYING THE PRINCIPLES OF FITNESS INTO YOUR CRF PROGRAM

Now that you have determined your level of CRF and commitment to begin working on your CRE, it is time to apply the principles of conditioning into your exercise program. This will help you to design a program that will guarantee improving your current level of CRE.

Warm Up Principle—Whatever aerobic activity you choose for your CRF program, you should warm up by using that or a similar activity at a lower intensity. For example, if you

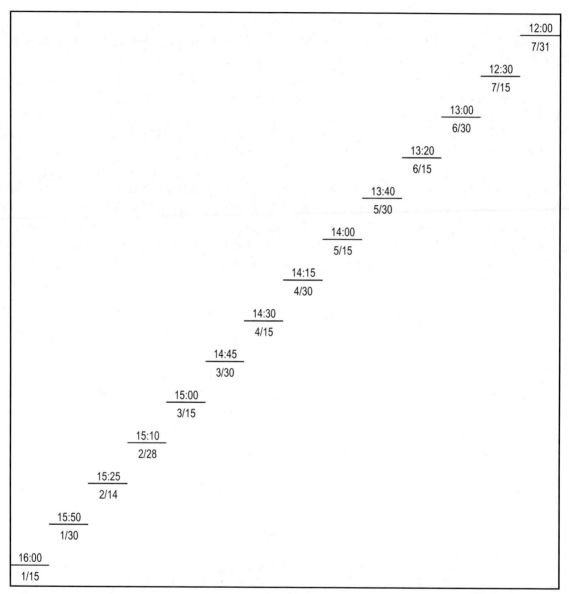

	12:00
	7/31

12:00
7/31

12:30
7/15

13:00
6/30

13:20
6/15

13:40
5/30

14:00
5/15

14:15
4/30

14:30
4/15

14:45
3/30

15:00
3/15

15:10
2/28

15:25
2/14

15:50
1/30

16:00
1/15

Stairway to Success... Marc ran 1.5 miles in 16:00. His goal is to be able to run 1.5 miles in 12:00. He knows this will not happen overnight and so he has set a long-term goal of being able to run 1.5 miles in 12:00 by 7/31. In the mean time, Marc has set several short-term goals that represents where he would like to be every two weeks. Each time Marc reaches his short-term goal, he will move up one step towards the next goal. If he does not reach his short-term goal, he can re-evaluate his actions and refer to Chapter 3 and BE SMAART.

Figure 6.6—Stairway to Success Based on 1.5-Mile Run

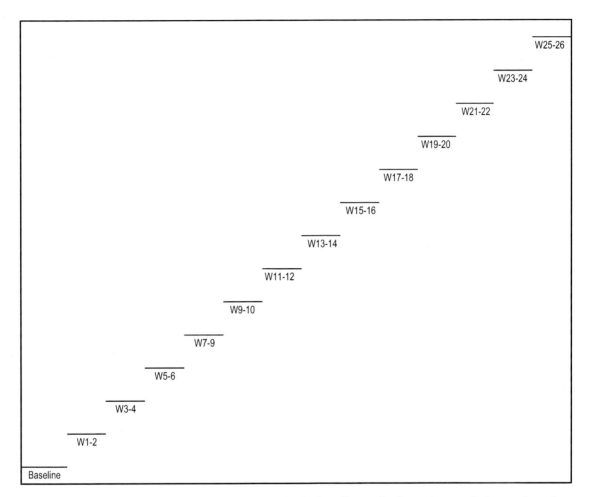

On the bottom of the stairs write down your present level of cardiovascular fitness in numerical terms (e.g., the number of continuous minutes you are exercising, distance covered, laps completed, etc. On the top of the stairs, write down what you would like to accomplish in 6 months. On the 2nd step to the bottom write down your first short-term goal and what you would like to accomplish within the next two weeks. When you reach your first short-term goal, proceed to the next step above and set your next short-term goal and so on until you reach your long-term goal. If at any time you are having difficulty reaching your short-term goals, return to Chapter 3 and review the section entitled "Exercise Barriers and Solutions.

Figure 6.6—My Stairway to Success

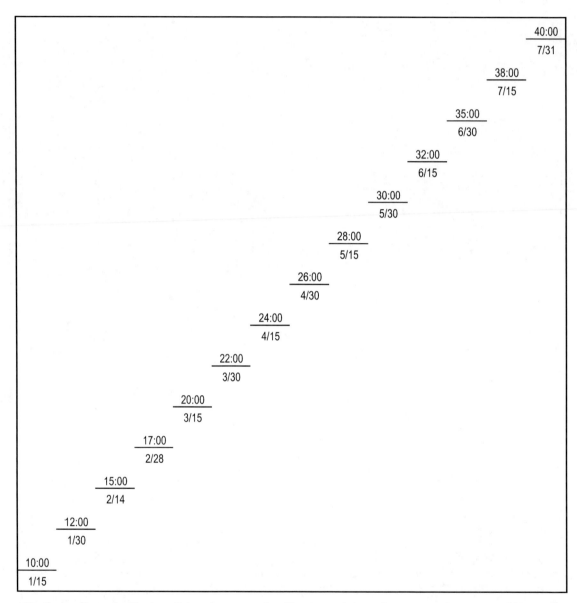

For those of you who like to walk here is an example of how to use your staircase to set short-term and long-term goals to improve your CRE through walking. Mae is a middle-aged woman who performed an informal CRE assessment of walking for 10 minutes on 1/15. Her long-term goal is to be able to walk for 40 minutes. Using the stairway to success, Mae has set goals to improve a few minutes every two weeks. By July 15, Mae will be able to reach her goal of walking 45 minutes (and she'll do it walking faster and more comfortably, too)!

Figure 6.6—Stairway to Success Based on 10-Minute Walk

plan to run, then warm up by walking briskly or jogging slowly for a few minutes. Once you feel your body is warmed up, you should then stretch for a few minutes. (See Chapter 8 for a list of flexibility exercises). This will get you ready to overload your cardiorespiratory endurance system.

Principle of Progression—If you review your exercise prescription for CRE, you will see systematic increases in frequency, intensity, and time. Time should be increased first, followed by either intensity or frequency (whichever motivates you more) since it is a lot easier to add on a few more minutes once you have gotten started than it is to find an extra day to exercise or make yourself go harder than you may be used to. Once you achieve 30 minutes of aerobic activity, you can plan to increase intensity (e.g., running a few seconds faster per mile; going from level 1 to 2 on the stationary bicycle; walking up and down hills) provided you stay within your target heart rate or add an extra day to your weekly workout schedule (provided it fits for you).

Principle of Individuality—Your CRE exercise prescription should be based on your level of CR fitness and commitment. Therefore, you should be prescribing aerobic activities that you like to do rather than what someone else wants you to do. In addition, the length of time you exercise and the intensity that you work at should be based on your own CRF level and not someone else. So stick to the exercise prescription that's designed just for you.

Principle of Recuperation—Make sure that you do not overdo it and give yourself enough rest to recuperate from your exercise overload. If your CRF level is low then you should rest at least one and preferably two days in between workouts. If your CRF level is moderate than you should rest every other day or every third day and if your CR fitness level is high, then you give yourself at least one, preferably two or even three of days rest if your workouts exceed 60 minutes. Most important, you should always listen to your body. It is always better to take the extra day's rest and feel ready for your next workout than to overwork yourself by exercising too many days in a row. See Figure 6.7 to see how you can incorporate the POR into your CRE program based on your present level of fitness and commitment to exercise 2-5 days per week.

Principle of Fun—You can make your CRE fun by incorporating activities that you like into your workout. So, if you like to listen to music then plan to use your CD, MP3, IPOD or radio while exercising. If you like to exercise with a partner than invite someone you know to exercise with you, join a gym or take an exercise class that appeals to you and set a goal to meet someone in class whose interests are similar to yours. If you like to exercise alone then find a quiet time in the gym or another place that is unoccupied to exercise. Once you blend what is fun for you into your exercise routine, you will look forward to and enjoy your workouts more.

Principle of Reversibility—Another way of stating the principle of reversibility is "use it or lose it." To avoid this principle you must stick to your exercise routine. Based on your level of commitment, you have decided how many days per week you will exercise. To keep you on task, you should write down your exercise schedule at the beginning of every week. Include day, time, length, activity, and facility into your day planner. Make a copy of it and place it in areas you frequent such as you car, office desk, locker, book bag and cell phone and stick to it. This way you won't have to worry about reversing what you have gained. You can use Figure 6.7 to help you.

CRE	Day 1	Day 2	Day 3	Day 4	Day 5	Day 6	Day 7
Low CRE 2✕ @ WK	EXERCISE	REST	REST	REST	EXERCISE	REST	REST
Low CRE 3✕ @ WK	EXERCISE	REST	EXERCISE	REST	EXERCISE	REST	REST
Low CRE 3✕ @ WK	EXERCISE	REST	REST	EXERCISE	REST	EXERCISE	REST
Mod CRE 3✕ @ WK	EXERCISE	REST	EXERCISE	REST	REST	EXERCISE	REST
Mod CRE 4✕ @ WK	EXERCISE	EXERCISE	REST	REST	EXERCISE	EXERCISE	REST
MOD CRE 4✕ @ WK	EXERCISE	REST	EXERCISE	EXERCISE	REST	EXERCISE	REST
High CRE 4✕ @ WK	EXERCISE	REST	EXERCISE	EXERCISE	REST	EXERCISE	REST
High CRE 5✕ @ WK	EXERCISE	EXERCISE	REST	EXERCISE	EXERCISE	REST	EXERCISE
High CRE 5✕ @ WK	EXERCISE	EXERCISE	EXERCISE	REST	EXERCISE	EXERCISE	REST

Figure 6.7—Incorporating the Principle of Recuperation into Your CRD Program

EVALUATING THE SUCCESS OF YOUR CRE PROGRAM

After your first week has been completed, it is now time to evaluate the success of your program. Did you reach your goals and exercise the number of times per week and minutes you committed to? Do you feel like you have more energy to exercise longer this week? Are the workouts getting a little easier? If you answered "YES" to all of these questions then you are ready to set new goals and move on to week 2. If you answered "NO" to any of these questions, it is time to identify what stopped you. Did you not reach your goals because the goals were too hard? If so, you should probably consider modifying your goals and make them a little less challenging and more realistic to your present CRF level and commitment. Perhaps you need to reduce the frequency by a day or the time by a few minutes. If you didn't reach your goal, but improved, you may just be a workout or two away so keep the same goal for this week, and write down a strategy for how you will reach your goal and stick to it. Perhaps you did not reach your goal because you were lazy or maybe you just didn't feel like you had the energy or desire to exercise? For whatever the reason, be aware that something "stopped you." Go back and review chapters 1 and 2 and determine what your plan of action is for next week. Incorporate specific strategies that will help you to stay on task and overcome what stopped you from reaching your goal in week 1. For example, write down your goal, the day(s) and time(s) you plan to exercise, what you will do, how long you will exercise for and how you will make your weekly workouts fun and something to look forward to. Remember, striving to reach your goal will only help you to enjoy the exercise more. Most important, it will remind you that you are committed to getting fit and staying fit for life.

Hopefully by now you realize how much control you have over your own progress. You determined how committed you were, what your level of CR fitness was and how much you were going to do in your CR workouts. Then you set a goal and evaluated its success. You came up with strategies to motivate yourself and stay on task and this should have enhanced your desire to continue exercising in week 2. If at any time you get stopped over the next few weeks and thereafter, all you need to do is re-examine your exercise prescription along with your perceptions of what stopped you. Then incorporate the strategies that make it more fun for you to continue and increase your commitment level. Once you make the commitment to have fun and improve, you will.

HOW TO PREVENT INJURIES WHILE ENGAGING IN CRE ACTIVITIES

The best way to deal with injuries is not to get them so follow these basic guidelines towards an injury free exercise routine.

1. *Consult Your Physician*—Before embarking on your CRE exercise program it is recommended that you consult your physician and discuss your desire to begin exercising especially if you are over 40 or have been diagnosed with certain preexisting conditions such as arthritis, asthma, tendonitis, heart condition, diabetes or epilepsy.

2. *Warm up first*—Before beginning your CR exercise, you should warm up your muscles in the same or similar way you plan to overload them just at a lower intensity. So, if you plan to go for a run, then you should warm up by walking and jogging lightly for a few minutes. Then, proceed to stretch your muscles and then you will be ready to run.

3. *Start out slowly*—Sometimes we want to get fit quick and overdo it by working out too intensely or too long. We may push ourselves beyond our normal capacity resulting in excessive soreness and possible injury. So start out slowly and listen to your body. If you are feeling excessive tension or you are getting out a breath then stop.

These are signs that you may be doing too much, too soon and increasing your chances of injury.

4. ***Select the right shoes***—Select a shoe that is designed for the exercise you plan to do. Try the shoe on in a store that specializes in the activities that you do. Then walk or jog on it to make sure that it feels comfortable. Inform the shoe specialist about your activities (e.g., walking, jogging, running, aerobic dance, bicycling, stair climbing, cross training), your planned exercise program (e.g., days per week, # of miles walking or running per week, etc), desired exercise facility (e.g., at home indoors, local gym, outdoor park), and surface being exercised on (e.g., treadmill, grass, track, street, hardwood floor). Examine your feet to see if you move straight or curved. You want to make sure that the shoe provides ample support and comfort in the working areas (e.g., heel, arch, ball, toe).

5. ***Cool down***—After you complete your workout, you body may be tired and your muscles may feel a little tight. Therefore you should cool down by walking slowly for a few minutes and then stretch out to alleviate any excessive tension created from your exercise overload.

6. ***Exercising in the Heat and Cold***—Exercising in hot weather can cause cramping, dehydration, heat exhaustion and heat stroke. To avoid this, you should make sure you are hydrated by drinking 10 to 20 ounces of water or a lightly salted liquid (e.g., Gatorade) about 15-30 minutes before exercising and every 15 minutes while exercising. In addition, on days that you are planning to exercise, you should increase your daily water/fluid consumption prior to exercising to make sure that you are appropriately hydrated. You should wear a hat or bandana to cover your head from the sun and your clothes should be light and comfortable. Avoid wearing sweat suits or long sleeved shirts as this will only increase body temperature. In cold weather, it is important to protect yourself from getting hypothermia or frostbite. Therefore, you should wear layers of clothing and protect exposed areas by keeping them covered. Wear gloves or mittens to cover your hands and thick athletic socks to keep your feet warm. Wear a hat to cover your head and ears and in extreme cold and windy conditions you should consider a scarf or ski mask to protect your face.

7. ***Learn proper form***—Sometimes injury can be caused by improper form. Therefore, before beginning your exercise program, become familiar with the proper form. If necessary, practice a few times and examine your form to see if it is correct. If you are having trouble then you should consider consulting with a qualified exercise professional as well as reading books that explain how to do the activities you have chosen properly.

This chapter has introduced cardiorespiratory endurance and explains the importance of being aerobically fit. A variety of CRE assessments, both formal and informal, based on one's level of CR fitness (low-moderate-high) are presented. In addition, exercise prescriptions are included and integrated based on CRF as well as level of commitment. Principles of fitness are reintroduced to help you improve your present level of CRF. Finally, strategies to prevent injuries are introduced to help you exercise safely.

REVIEW QUESTIONS

1. Define cardiorespiratory endurance.

2. Explain the differences between a fit vs. an unfit heart

3. List at least eight physical and psychological benefits of being CR fit.

4. What is the purpose of assessing your CR fitness?

5. List three ways you can formally assess your CRE and explain the strengths and limitations of each.

6. What is an informal assessment and explain when it is beneficial to use this methodology to assess CR fitness?

7. Define the four components of an exercise prescription and include an example of each.

8. Discuss two ways you measure the exercise intensity for CRE activities.

9. Define three levels of exercise commitment and explain how you can increase a low commitment level to a high commitment level.

10. Explain the benefits of setting SMAART goals for your CR fitness program.

11. Discuss how you would determine if your CR fitness program was successful?

12. Describe how you can incorporate the principles of progression, specificity, individuality, warm up, recuperation, reversibility, and fun into a CR fitness program.

13. What strategies can you incorporate to reduce and prevent the chances of injury?

LAB ASSIGNMENT 6.1

Questions 1-9 should be answered prior to beginning your CR fitness program.

1. How committed are you to improving your CR fitness over the next 4 weeks? If you have a low level of commitment, what strategies will you incorporate to increase your level of commitment?

2. What are your SMART goals for improving your CRE over the next 4 weeks?
   A. _____
   B. _____
   C. _____

3. Using the Stairway to Success, convert your SMAART goals into stairway goals over the next four weeks.

                                                        _____

                                        _____

                        _____

        _____

4. Develop an exercise prescription to improve your CR fitness over the next four weeks.

	Week 1	Week 2	Week 3	Week 4
F				
I				
T				
T				

5. Explain how you will be progressing in CR fitness from weeks 1 to 4?

6. Describe how you plan to incorporate the principle of recuperation into your CR fitness program?

7. What do you plan to do to satisfy the warm up principle?

8. What strategies are you considering to incorporate the principle of fun?

9. What strategies do you have planned to avoid the principle of reversibility?

Questions 10-14 should be answered at the conclusion of each week.

10. Explain how you have been overloading your CR endurance system from Weeks 1-2-3-4?

11. How has your recuperation time changed from weeks' 1-4?

12. How successful were you in avoiding the principle of reversibility?

13. How much have your improved from weeks' 1-4?

14. Did you have fun while working on your CR fitness? If so, explain the strategies that you used to have fun? If you did not have fun, explain what you plan to do to make your CR workouts more fun next week (e.g., music, exercising with a partner, etc).

REFERENCES

American College of Sports Medicine.com (2005).

Blair, S.N., Kohl III, W., Paffenbarger, Jr., R.S., Clark, D.G., Cooper, K.H., & Gibbons, L.W. (1998). Physical fitness and all-cause mortality: A prospective study of healthy men and women. *Journal of the American Medical Association, 262*, 2395-2401.

Borg G. (1998). Borg's perceived exertion and pain scales. Champaign, IL, Human Kinetics.

Fahey, T.D., Insel, P.M., & Roth, W.T. (2005). Applying the FITT Equation pp 68 in Fit and well: Core concepts and labs in physical fitness and wellness. 6th edition, McGraw Hill. Griest, J.H., Klein, M.H., Eischens, R.R., & Faris, J.T. (1978). Running out of depression. *Physician and Sportsmedicine, 6*, 49-56.

Lox, C.L., Martin Ginis, K.A., Petruzzello, S.J. (2006). Health-related quality of life and exercise, pp, 389-415, in C.L. Lox, K.A. Martin Ginis, & S.J. Petruzzello, *The Psychology of exercise: Integrating theory and practice,* (pp. 389-415) 2nd edition, Holcomb Hathaway Publishers

Morgan, W.P. (1997). Physical activity and mental health. Washington, DC: Taylor & Francis. Morgan, W.P., & Goldston, S.E. (1987). Exercise and mental health. Washington, DC: Hemisphere.

Pate, R.R., Pratt, M., Blain, S.N., Haskell, W.L., Macera, C.A., Bouchard, C., Buckner, D., Ettinger, W., Heath, G. W., King, A.C., Kriska, A., Leon, A.S., Marcus, B.H., Morris, J., Paffenbarger, R.S., Jr., Patrick, P., Pollock, M.L., Rippe, J.M., Sallis, J., & Wilmore, J.H. (1995). Physical activity and public health. *Journal of the American Medical Association, 273,* 402-407.

Pollack, M.L., Rippe, J.M., Sallis, J., & Wilmore, J.H. (1995). Physical activity and public health. *Journal of the American Medical Association, 273,* 402-407.

Ryan, A.J. (1983). Exercise is medicine. Physician and Sportsmedicine, 11, 10. United States Department of Health and Human Services, 1996. Physical activity and health: A report of the Surgeon General. Report DHHS publication no. (PH5) 017-023-00196-5. Atlanta: U.S. Department of Health and Human Services, Centers for Disease Control and Prevention, National Center for Chronic Disease Prevention and Health Promotion.

United States Department of Health and Human Services, 1996. Physical activity and health: A report of the Surgeon General. Report DHHS publication no. (PH5) 017-023-00196-5, Atlanta, U.S. Department of Health and Human Services, Center for Disease Control and Prevention, National Center for Chronic Disease Prevention and Health Promotion.

APPENDIX 6A
WEEKLY GOAL SHEET FOR CRE

Name _____ Date: _____

Select 1-2 goals that will help you improve your CRE. Write down your goal(s) in the "Goal(s) Selected" column next to the category of goal that you have selected. Using the 7 Day Chart down below, record each day's workout next to the appropriate activity and under the actual day. After the week is up, add up your total workout performances and put them in the "Performance Results" column. If you achieved you weekly goal, mark an "A" across from your goal category in the "Achieved" column. If you did not reach your goal, mark an "NA" across from you goal category and under the "Not Achieved" column.

Category of Goals to Select From	Goal(s) Selected	Performance Results	Achieved = A	Not Achieved = NA
CRE Goals				
Frequency of Weekly Workouts				
Time in Minutes Exercised for Week				
Activity Selected				
Run / Walk				
Bicycle				
Elyptical				
Rowing				
Stairmaster				
Other				

	Day 1	Day 2	Day 3	Day 4	Day 5	Day 6	Day 7
CRE							
Run/Walk							
Bicycle							
Elyptical							
Rowing							
Stairmaster							
Other							

Appendix 6B
Stairway to CRE Success

6-7 Month Stairway

10-20 WEEK STAIRWAY TO SUCCESS

Chapter 7

Developing an Exercise Prescription for Muscular Fitness

OBJECTIVES

After this chapter, you will be able to:

- Define muscular fitness and distinguish between muscular strength & muscular endurance
- Understand the benefits of being muscularly fit
- Assess your muscular fitness safely
- Develop an exercise prescription for muscular fitness
- Determine your level of commitment to being muscularly fit
- Spice up your muscular fitness program
- Incorporate principles of fitness into your muscular fitness program
- Set S.M.A.A.R.T. goals that motivate you to work on your muscular fitness
- Evaluate the success of your muscular fitness program
- Learn how to minimize and prevent injuries while engaging in muscular fitness activities

Over the past thirty years, the popularity of weight training has grown tremendously with more men and women participating in weight training programs in both public and private exercise facilities than ever before. At one time, however, weight training was viewed as a masculine activity, designed to help people "bulk up" or increase their muscular size. This decreased the interest for many people, specifically women who were motivated to tone their muscles and improve their fitness yet not increase their muscular size. Consequently, there were less women enrolling in weight training classes and participating in the weight rooms of local exercise facilities. While this common misconception still exists today, more and more people have become educated about the benefits of weight training. Specifically, they have learned that hormonal differences between men and women do not allow women to gain muscular size in the same way that men do. Men have more testosterone, which is a growth-producing hormone and one of the main factors in producing increases in muscular size. So not only will women not bulk up, those who choose to participate in weight training will notice better shape and tone to their muscles (Hesson, 2006). Just remember, weight training is equally beneficial for men and women. In this chapter, you will learn how to assess your muscular strength and endurance and design a muscular fitness (MF) program that clearly meets your needs (e.g., tone, shape and define your muscles, improve strength, build muscle and increase muscular size). You will become an educated consumer and learn how to weight train safely and productively so that you can do what is best for you! Ready, Set, Lift your fingers to the next page and let's get started!

WHAT IS MUSCULAR FITNESS?

Muscular fitness consists of two components: muscular strength and muscular endurance. *Muscular strength* is the ability of the muscles to generate maximum force. For example, you are working on your muscular strength when you lift weights or carry objects heavy enough that you can only hold them for a short period of time or lift for a few reps before your muscle(s) fatigue. *Muscular endurance* is the capability of a muscle to produce submaximal force repeatedly over time by contracting the muscles or holding a contraction for a long time. An example of muscular endurance is performing many repetitions of an exercise (e.g., 20 crunches) or holding packages for several minutes. While muscular strength and endurance are interrelated, training for each is somewhat different. Specifically, if you want to develop muscular strength, then you will be lifting heavier weights fewer times (e.g., 2-8 reps per set, 70%-90% of your 1 rep max) and if you want to develop muscular endurance, then you will lift lighter weights for more repetitions (12-20 reps at 50%- 60% of your one-rep max). Finally, if you want to develop both muscular strength and endurance, then you will be somewhere in the middle and you will be lifting a moderate amount of weight for 8-12 reps (60%-70% of your 1 rep max) per set.

BENEFITS OF MUSCULAR FITNESS TRAINING (MFT)

There are many benefits to MFT. The key is to find the one(s) that attracts you most towards getting started and improving your MF. Listed below are 11 different benefits that can be achieved from MFT.

1. *Reduced rate of injury*—As your muscles get stronger, they are more resistant to fatigue and will not break down as easily. This will decrease your susceptibility to getting injured.

2. ***Reduced rate of low back problems***—One of the main causes of back problems is having weak back and abdominal muscles. MFT will help to strengthen these areas and reduce and possibly even prevent back problems.

3. ***Reduced risk of Osteoporosis***—Improving strength with increase bone density and make you less prone to bone fractures and weak bones.

4. ***Weight control***—As you build up and shape your muscles, your metabolism will increase which will help to increase weight loss and maintain the proper body weight.

5. ***Improved athletic performance***—Many sport teams employ strength and conditioning coaches to help athletes build muscular strength and endurance, speed and power which aid in improving athletic performance across a wide variety of sports.

6. ***Improved recreational performance***—All recreational activities require some degree of muscular fitness. When you have poor levels of either muscular strength or endurance, it limits your ability to perform well in many activities (e.g., walking, jogging, jumping, hiking, swimming, racquet sports, basketball, baseball, bowling, volleyball, football) just to name a few. Increasing your muscular fitness can improve performance in these areas and increase your enjoyment, too.

7. ***Better quality of life***—As a result of being muscularly fit, you will be able to accomplish more on a daily basis without getting tired (e.g., lifting heavy objects; carrying your books around all day; walking up and down stairs). More energy means more productivity which can also improve the quality of your life.

8. ***Increase self-esteem & self-confidence***—Your confidence will increase as you see improvements in your workout. Yesterday's hard workout becomes today's easier workout. You will challenge yourself to conquer new and exciting goals (e.g., getting to the next weight, adding a few more reps, learning a new exercise) as your early hesitation about muscular fitness training has been replaced with a strong belief that you can accomplish whatever you set your mind and body towards.

9. ***Looking better***—Toned muscles take up less space than body fat. Therefore, working on your MFT will not only tone and define your muscles, it will make you look and feel better about yourself.

10. ***Manage stress and anxiety better***—Making the commitment to build up your MF and challenging yourself to improve will help to take your mind off of daily stressors. In addition, when you see and feel the results, it will decrease anxiety that often confronts you when you are not taking good care of yourself. In chapter 12 you will learn more about identifying your stressors and using exercises as a way to cope with and eventually get rid of unwanted stress in your life.

11. ***Improve health and slow down the aging process***—As you improve your muscular fitness, your health will improve, too. Your muscles will become stronger and the natural aging process will slow down which can prevent certain illnesses from occurring. What a great feeling to get older and feel younger.

ASSESSING YOUR MUSCULAR FITNESS

Although muscular strength and endurance are related, the way they are measured and trained for is different. This section provides information for how to assess your muscular strength and endurance.

Assessing Muscular Strength

The most common way to assess your muscular strength is with a one-rep max test. This involves lifting as much weight as you can one time. For example, say you want to see how strong your legs are. You go over to the leg press and lift 200 lbs. If you can do it more than one time, then you would continue to raise the weight until you could no longer complete one rep. The most weight that you can successfully lift one time represents your max test results and your true muscular strength in that area.

Procedure for the One Rep Max Test

1. Familiarize yourself with the equipment (proper sitting position, appropriate range of motion).
2. Select 1-2 exercises that work the major muscle groups of the body. (See Figure 7.1)
3. Learn proper form by practicing a few times. If performing the max test is part of a class requirement (e.g., weight training, physical conditioning, fitness for life, then one class should be devoted to practicing and the next class to max testing. See Figure 7.2 to see correct and incorrect form for resistance training exercises.
4. Have a spotter with you to make sure you are performing each exercise properly.
5. Warm up first by lifting a light amount of weight for 8-12 reps.
6. Proceed to lifting a weight for one rep.
7. If successful, continue to lift the highest amount of weight that you can for one rep
8. Record your results on your Muscular Fitness Assessment Form (See Figure 7.2)

Chest	Back	Shoulders
Bench Press	Lat Pull Down	Shoulder Press
Seated Fly	Low Row	Rear Deltoid
	High Row/T Bar	
Legs	**Triceps**	**Biceps**
Leg Press	Tricep Pull Down	Preacher Curls
Leg Curl	Tricep Extension	
Leg Extension		
Hack Squat		

Figure 7.1—Exercises to Max On

Exercises to Max On

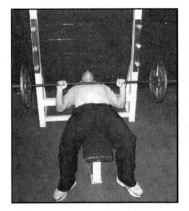 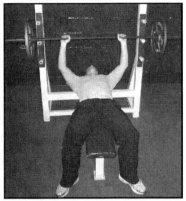

Bench Press Resting   **Bench Press Exertion**

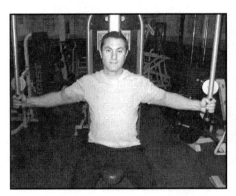 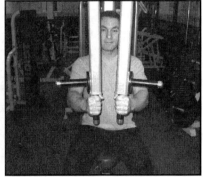

Seated Fly Resting   **Seated Fly Exertion**

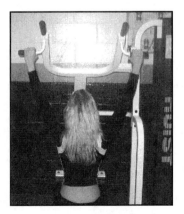 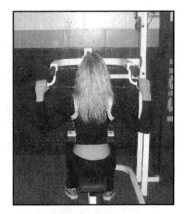

Lat Pulldown Resting   **Lat Pulldown Exertion**

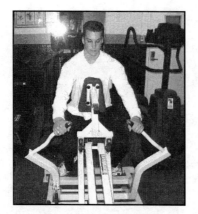

Low Row Resting

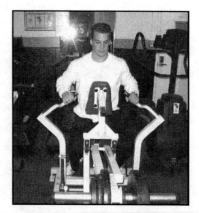

Low Row Exertion

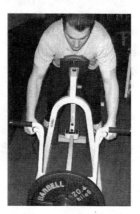

T Bar Resting

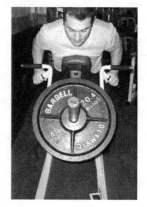

T Bar Exertion

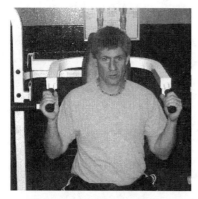

Shoulder Press Down Resting

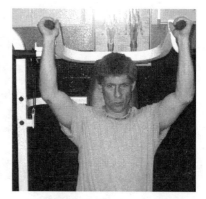

Shoulder Press Down Exertion

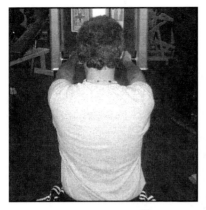
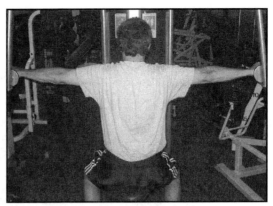

Rear Deltoid Resting   **Rear Deltoid Exertion**

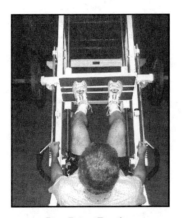
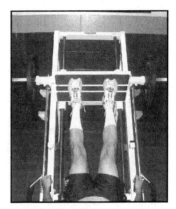

Leg Press Resting   **Leg Press Exertion**

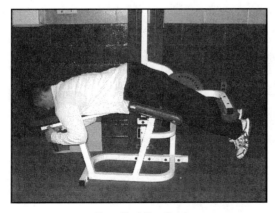
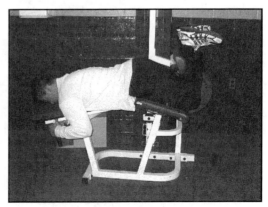

Leg Curl Resting   **Leg Curl Exertion**

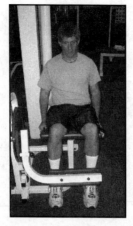 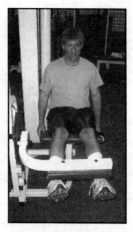

Leg Extension Resting   **Leg Extension Exertion**

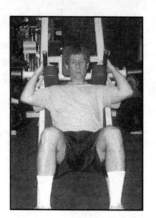 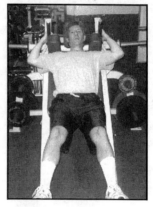

Hack Squat Resting   **Hack Squat Exertion**

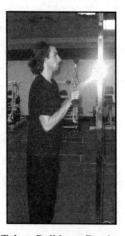 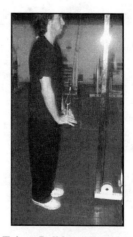

Tricep Pulldown Resting   **Tricep Pulldown Exertion**

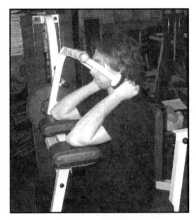

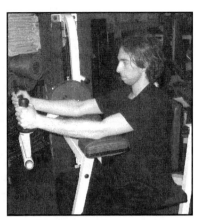

Tricep Extension Resting   **Tricep Extension Exertion**

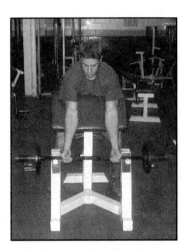

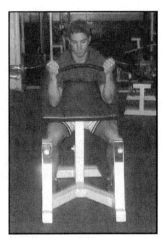

Preacher Curl Resting   **Preacher Curl Exertion**

Assessing Muscular Endurance

Muscular endurance can be assessed by performing the maximum number of repetitions of a submaximal resistance or by the length of time a person can hold a contraction (e.g., flexed arm hang) (Hoeger & Hoeger, 2005). For example: If you maxed 100 lbs on the bench press, how many reps of 50 lbs (50% of your max) can you perform? How many push ups can you do or how long can you hang on a chin up bar. Some of the more popular exercises to assess your muscular endurance include: push ups, sit ups and curl ups. (Use Figure 7.2 to record your results on your Muscular Fitness Assessment Form).

	Pre Test		Mid-Test		Post-Test	
	Max Sub Max		*Max Sub Max*		*Max Sub Max*	
Chest						
Bench Press						
Seated Fly						
Chest Press						
Back						
Lat Pull Down						
Low Row						
High Row/T Bar						
Shoulders						
Shoulder Press						
Rear Deltoid						
Legs						
Leg Press						
Leg Curl						
Leg Extension						
Hack Squat						
Triceps						
Tricep Extension						
Tricep Pulldown						
Bicep						
Barbell Curl						
Preacher Curl						
Arm Curl						
Upper body						
Pushups						
Flex Arm Hang						
Abdominals						
Sit ups or Curl Ups						
Abdominal Machine						

For max tests—record the highest amount of weight lifted for one repetition ***For sub max tests***—record the total number of repetitions achieved ***Flexed Arm Hang***—record the total number of seconds held on the chin up bar

Figure 7.2—Muscular Fitness Assessment Form

SAFE AND UNSAFE WAYS TO LIFT WEIGHTS

Although lifting weights has been around for many years across a variety of settings (e.g., school, military, sports, exercise facilities, local Y), proper form and techniques have not always been practiced. Consequently, many individuals have developed bad habits and use incorrect form resulting in a higher risk of injuries and decrease in productivity. Figure 7.3 includes a list of common weight training exercises along with the common mistake and correction.

Exercise	Common Mistake	Correction
Bench Press	Arching the back—creates undue stress on the lower and central parts of the back;	Place feet flat on the floor and keep back flat on the bench with knees flexed to insure back stays flat throughout lift;
Lat Pull-down	Arching back/leaning backwards—creates stress on the lower back;	Keep back straight; Avoid using machines that place handles in the back of the neck and instead use machines that place handles in the front of the chest;
Seated Row	Arching back on the exertion phase—causes stress on the lower back;	Lean forward on the resting phase and keep back straight up on the exertion phase as the handles reach abdominal section;
Shoulder Press	Leaning and tilting head forward creates stress on the neck & upper back;	Keep hands in an upright position with head and back aligned straight;
Leg Press	Moving too fast and locking knees—causes excessive strain on the knees	Proceed slowly on the resting phases to the point where your knees are slightly bent and never straightened;
Tricep Extension	Locking elbows—causes excessive strain on the elbow	Proceed slowly on the exertion phase to the point where your arms are almost fully extended keeping elbows bent slightly bent;
Tricep Pulldown	Raising bar above chest height causing elbows to move away from sides of body; this allows your chest to help you lift the weight, thus creating reduced work for the triceps;	Keep elbows next to your sides with no space in between; bring bar up slowly on the resting phase to chest height and not higher;
Bicep Curl	Arching backwards on the exertion phase in order to complete the full range of motion;	Keep back straight and avoid leaning forward or backward;
Sit Up	Interlocking hands behind neck	Place fingertips behind ears or cross arms in front of body with no space between elbows and body
Crunches	Knees over chest	Knees over hips

Figure 7.3— Common Mistakes and Corrections of Popular Resistance Training Exercises

Common Mistakes and Corrections

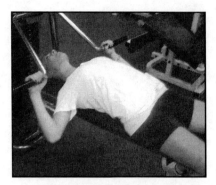

Bench Press Arching Back

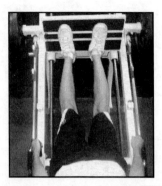

Leg Press Knees Locked

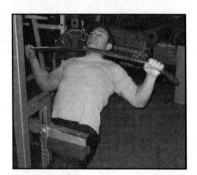

Lat Pulldown Arching Back

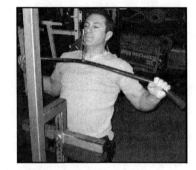

Lat Pulldown Correct Form

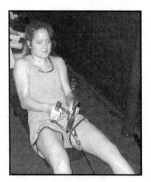

**Seated Row
Arching Back**

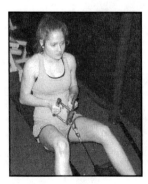

**Seated Row
Correct Form**

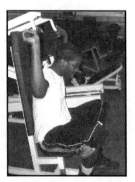

**Shoulder Press
Tilting Head Forward**

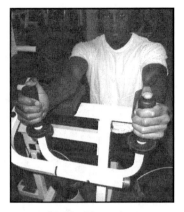

**Tricep Extension
Locking Elbows**

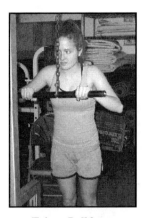

**Tricep Pulldown
Elbows away from Body**

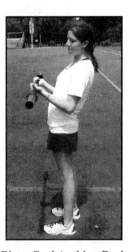

Bicep Curl Arching Back

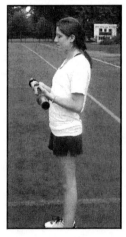

Bicep Curl Correct Form

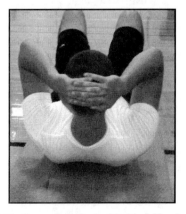

Sit Up finger Interlocked behind Head

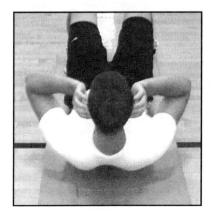

Sit Up Correct Form

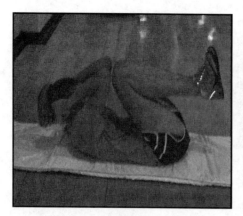
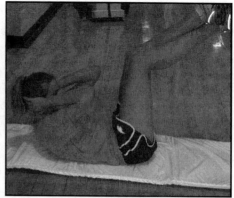

Crunches Knees Too Close to Chest   **Crunches Correct Form**

See figure 7.1 for correct form for bench press, leg press, shoulder press, tricep extension and tricep pulldown.

DEVELOPING AN EXERCISE PRESCRIPTION FOR MUSCULAR FITNESS (MF)

The four components of an exercise prescription for MF are identical to the ones introduced in Chapter 6 for CRE (F-I-T-T). However, the way you measure each component for MF is slightly different than for CRE.

Frequency—There are two ways to determine frequency of a MFT program: (1) days per week you will work on MF and (2) days per week you will work on a specific muscle group. It is recommended that you work on each of the major muscle groups 1× per week over a 2-5 day period. This will allow your muscles enough time to recuperate after being overloaded.

Intensity—Since MFT does not focus on overloading the heart, checking your HR will not define how hard you are working. Therefore, intensity is measured by either percent max being used and/or completion of the desired number of reps. For example, if you want to work on muscular strength and endurance and you have completed your max test, you would using between 60-70 percent of your max. So if you maxed 100 lbs on a bench press, you would be working out with 60 or 70 lbs.

Intensity can also be determined by the number of desired reps achieved. For example, if you want to tone your muscles, you would be completing 12-15 reps per set. If you achieve 15 reps in a given set, then you should raise the weight on the next set. If you cannot achieve 12 reps, then the weight is too heavy and you should lower the weight. See Table 7.1 for a description of proper intensity using both percent max and desired number of reps for muscular fitness training.

Table 7.1
Determining Proper Intensity Using Percent Max and Desired Number of Reps

Type of Training	% Max	Desired Range of Reps	Recommendations
Muscular Strength	70% or greater	2-8	Increase weight once 8 reps are achieved in a set
Muscular Strength and Endurance	60% –70%	8-12	Increase weight once 12 reps are achieved in a set and decrease weight on next set if 8 reps cannot be achieved
Muscular Endurance "Body Toning"	50%–60%	12-15	Increase weight once 15 reps are achieved in a set and decrease weight if 12 reps cannot be achieved

Time—Typically, you would measure time by how long you workout (e.g., minutes, hours). However, with MFT, minutes would not be appropriate measures of time since the majority of time spent during MFT is sitting down or resting in between sets. Moreover, claiming you worked on MF for an hour doesn't tell you what you have accomplished. Therefore, you should measure time by answering five basic questions:

1. What body parts will you work on today?

2. How many exercises will you do for each body part?

3. How many sets will you do for each exercise?

4. What is your range of reps for each exercise that you plan to do (e.g., 2-8, 8-12, 12-15)?

5. How much time will you take off in between sets?

For example, let's say Josh wants to work on his legs and shoulders today. He will select three exercises for each body part and perform 2 sets of each exercise. Since he wants to work his strength, he will be striving to lift 2-8 reps per set and take 90 seconds off in between sets to recuperate. His workout is complete when he finishes the last rep of his last set from his last exercise.

Type—addresses all of the exercises you will consider doing for each of the major muscle groups. Of course, the place you choose to work on your MF can play a significant role in the exercises you select (e.g., equipment available, crowdedness of facility). However, there is no one specific exercise that you have to do in order to improve a specific body part(s) and therefore it is a good idea to have a list of different exercises to choose from (e.g., free weight, machines). See Figure 7.4 for a list of the muscular fitness exercises to choose from.

CHEST	BACK	SHOULDERS
Dumbbell Bench Press	Barbell Row	Barbell Upright Row
Universal Bench Press	One-arm Dumbbell Row	Dumbbell Upright Row
Decline Bench Press	Incline Dumbbell Row	Front Raises
Incline Bench Press	Lat Pulldown (See Exercise 3)	Lateral Raises
Decline Dumbbell Press	Low Row (See Exercise 4)	Bent Over Lateral Raises
Bent Arm Dumbbell Flys	High Row (See Exercise 5)	Shoulder Shrugs
Bent Arm Decline Flys	Hack Squat (See Exercise 6)	Dumbbell Press
Incline Dumbbell Flys		Shoulder Press (See Exercise 6)
Dumbbell Chest Press		Rear Deltoid (See Exercise 7)
Bench Press (See Fig 7.1 Exercise 1)		
Seated Fly (See Exercise 2)		

TRICEPS	BICEPS	LEGS
One Arm Tricep Extension	Barbell Curl	Dumbbell Lunges
Two Arm Tricep Extension	Hammer Curl	Wall Sit
Dip Machine	Seated Curl	Abductor
Bench Dips	Concentrations	Adductor
Lying Tricep Extension	Incline Dumbbell Curl	Leg Press (See Exercise 8)
Tricep Press	Alternating Dumbbell Curl	Leg Curl (See Exercise 9)
Lying Tricep Dumbbell Extension	Preacher Curl	Leg Extension (See Exercise 10)
Kickbacks	(See Exercise 14)	Hack Squat (See Exercise 11)
Tricep Pulldown (See Exercise 12)		
Tricep Extension (See Exercise 13)		

ABDOMINALS

Seeing Through Your Legs
Shoulders to the Sky
12-18's
Crossovers
Bicycles
SETK (Same Elbow to Knee)
Opposite Leg Raise
Sit Up
Touch My Toes Above
Reach My Toes
Climb the Rope
Crunches
Crossover Crunches
Standing Twists
Seated Twists
Squeeze Me

All large muscle group and upper body exercises (chest, back, shoulders, tricep, bicep, legs) are performed with free weights using barbells or dumbbells unless listed as a machine. Abdominal exercises are performed using own body weight to create resistance.

Figure 7.4—Muscular Fitness Exercises to Choose From

Chest Exercises

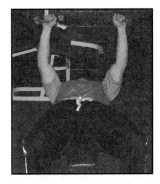
Dumbbell Bench Press

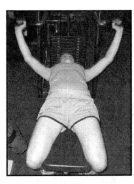
Universal Bench Press

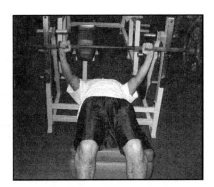
Decline Bench Press

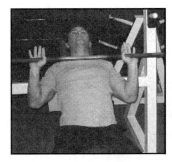
Incline Bench Press

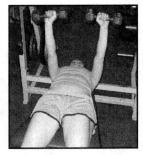
**Decline Dumbbell
Bench Press**

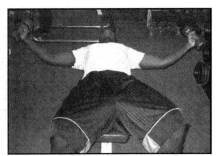
Bent Arm Dumbbell Flys

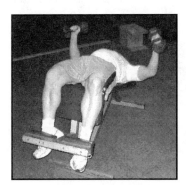
Bent Arm Decline Flys

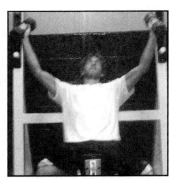
Incline Dumbbell Flys

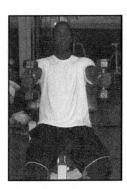
Dumbbell Chest Press

Back Exercises

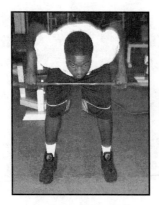
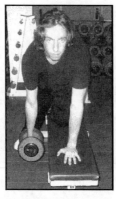
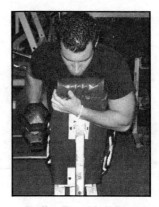

Barbell Row   **One-Arm Dumbbell Row**   **Incline Dumbbell Row**

Shoulder Exercises

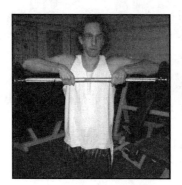
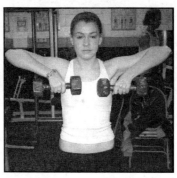
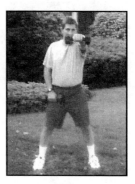

Barbell Upright Row   **Dumbbell Upright Row**   **Front Raise**

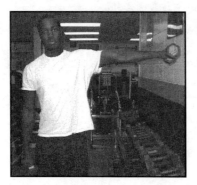
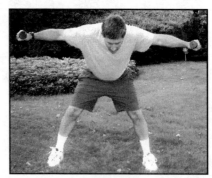

Lateral Raise   **Bent Over Lateral Raise**

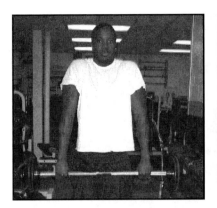

Shoulder Shrug

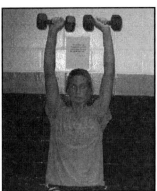

Dumbbell Press

Tricep Exercises

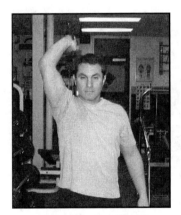

**One Arm Dumbbell
Tricep Extension**

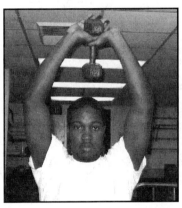

**Two Arm Dumbbell
Tricep Extension**

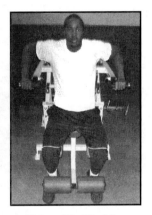

Tricep Dip Machine

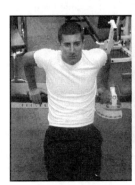

Bench Dips

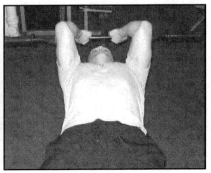

Lying Tricep Extension

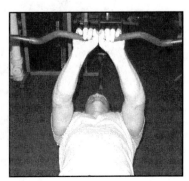

Tricep Press

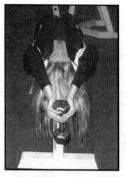 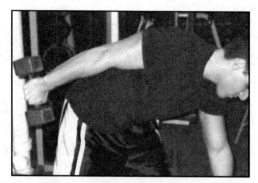

Lying Tricep Dumbbell Extensions   **Kickbacks**

Bicep Exercises

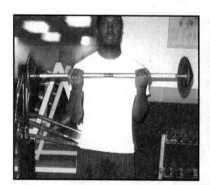 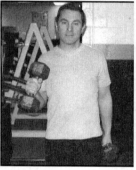 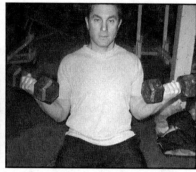

Barbell Curl   **Hammer Curl**   **Seated Curl**

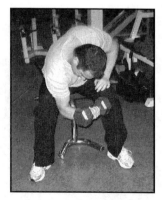 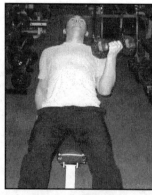 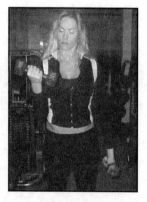

Concentrations   **Incline Dumbbell Curl**   **Alternating Dumbbell Curl**

Leg Exercises

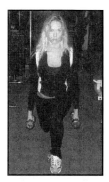
Dumbbell Lunges

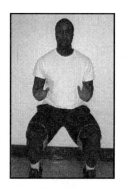
Wall Sit

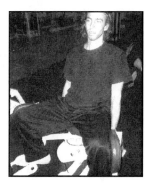
Abductor

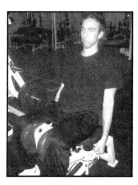
Abductor

Abdominal Exercises

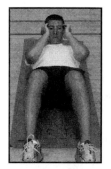
**Seeing through
Your Legs**

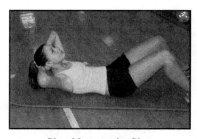
Shoulders to the Sky

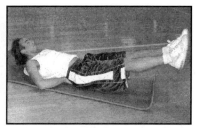
12-18's

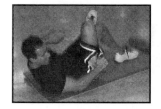
Cross Overs

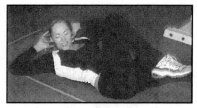
Bicycles

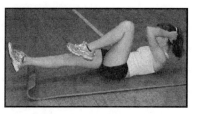
SETK Same Elbow to Knee

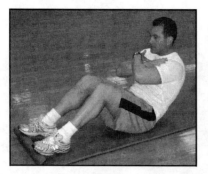

Sit Up

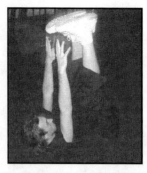

Touch My Toes Above

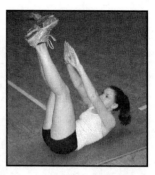

Toe Touches

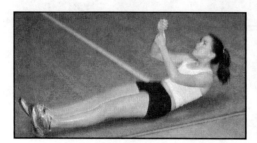

Climb the Rope

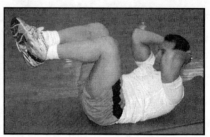

Crunches

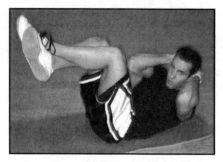

Cross Over Crunches

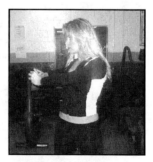

Standing Twists

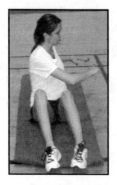

Seated Twists

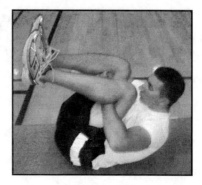

Squeeze Me

How Many Days Should I Work on Muscular Fitness?

Ideally, it is recommended that you work on MF two to four times per week. This will give you an opportunity to sufficiently overload each of the major muscle groups while also providing enough days in the week to rest and recuperate so you can be ready for next week's workouts. However, for those individuals who are only willing to commit one day per week towards working on MF, acknowledge yourself for getting started. While you may not see significant improvements from one day per week of training, you will see some modest gains (e.g., performing more reps of the same weight, increasing weight, adding sets, adding exercises; slight increases in body shaping and strength) in the first few weeks and this progress can motivate you more towards considering on working at least one more day per week and possibly more in the near future. Once you do find that second day, you will notice that the benefits will far outweigh the limitations. However, in the mean time, you can use Table 7.2 for your one-day muscular fitness program.

What Do I Want to Accomplish?

Muscular strength programs are designed for those individuals whose primary goals are to get stronger and increase their muscular size. Muscular endurance programs are designed for those individuals who want to tone, shape and define their muscles without increasing muscular size. The combination programs are designed for those individuals who want a little bit of everything (increase MS and ME, tone and define muscles while also increasing somewhat in muscular size).

Guidelines for Working on Muscular Fitness

When working on muscular strength, you will be lifting more weight for less reps and since the intensity is greater more recuperation time in between sets of work is generally needed. Tables 7.2–7.6 display three different muscular fitness programs that center on your level of muscular fitness (e.g., beginner-intermediate-advanced) and the number of days per week you are committing towards working on your muscular strength from one to five days.

Since advanced MF training requires more work on each of the major muscle groups than beginner or intermediate programs (e.g., more exercises, more sets), it cannot be achieved in one day per week of training. Therefore, it has been omitted from the one-day MF training program.

Table 7.2
Training for Muscular Fitness One Day Per Week

	Week 1	Week 2	Week 3	Week 4
F	**1**	**1**	**1**	**1**
I-MS	70%-90% of max or 2-8 reps per set	70%-90% of max or 2-8 reps per set	70%-90% of max or 2-8 reps per set	70%-90% of max or 2-8 reps per set
I-CB	60%-70% of max or 8-12 reps per set	60%-70% of max or 8-12 reps per set	60%-70% of max or 8-12 reps per set	60%-70% of max or 8-12 reps per set
I-ME	50%-60% of max or 12-15 reps per set	50%-60% of max or 12-15 reps per set	50%-60% of max or 12-15 reps per set	50%-60% of max or 12-15 reps per set
T-	***Beginners*** 1-2 exercises for each of the 6 major muscle groups & 1-set of each; 6-9 sets total; ***Intermediate*** 1-2 exercises for each of the 6 major muscle groups & 1-2 sets of each; 10-12 sets total;	***Beginners*** 1-2 exercises for each of the 6 major muscle groups & 1-2 sets of each; 9-12 sets total; ***Intermediate*** 1-3 exercises for each of the 6 major muscle groups & 2 sets of each; 12-15 sets total;	***Beginners*** 1-2 exercises for each of the 6 major muscle groups; 1-2 sets of each; 12-14 sets total; ***Intermediate*** 1-3 exercises for each of the 6 major muscle groups & 2 sets of each; 15-18 sets of each;	***Beginners*** 2 exercises for each of the 6 major muscle groups; 1-2 sets of each; 14-16 sets total; ***Intermediate*** 1-3 exercises for each of the 6 major muscle groups & 2 sets of each; 18-20 sets of each;
T See Figure 7.4 for a list of exercises to choose from				

MS—Muscular Strength; CB – Combination of Muscular Strength & Endurance; ME – Muscular Endurance

Table 7.3
Training for Muscular Fitness Two Days Per Week

	Week 1	Week 2	Week 3	Week 4
F	2	2	2	2
I-MS	70%-90% of max or 2-8 reps per set	70%-90% of max or 2-8 reps per set	70%-90% of max or 2-8 reps per set	70%-90% of max or 2-8 reps per set
I-CB	60%-70% of max or 8-12 reps per set	60%-70% of max or 8-12 reps per set	60%-70% of max or 8-12 reps per set	60%-70% of max or 8-12 reps per set
I-ME	50%-60% of max or 12-15 reps per set	50%-60% of max or 12-15 reps per set	50%-60% of max or 12-15 reps per set	50%-60% of max or 12-15 reps per set
T-	*Beginners* 2 exercises per body part; 1-2 sets per exercise; *Intermediate* 3 exercises per body part; 2 sets per exercise; *Advanced* 4 exercises per body part; 3 sets per exercise	*Beginners* 2-3 exercises per body part; 1-2 sets per exercise; *Intermediate* 3-4 exercises per body part; 2-3 sets per exercise *Advanced* 4-5 exercises per body part; 3-4 sets per exercise	*Beginners* 3 exercises per body part; 2 sets per exercise; *Intermediate* 4 exercises per body part; 3 sets per exercise *Advanced* 5 exercises per body part; 4 sets per exercise;	*Beginners* 3 exercises per body part 2-3 sets per exercise; *Intermediate* 4-5 exercises per body part; 3 sets per exercise *Advanced* 5 exercises per body part; 4-5 sets per exercise
T	Day 1 Chest-Triceps-Shoulders Day 2 Back-Biceps-Legs	Day 1 Chest-Triceps-Shoulders Day 2 Back-Biceps-Legs	Day 1 Chest-Back-Shoulders Day 2 Legs-Triceps-Biceps	Day 1 Chest-Back-Shoulders Day 2 Legs-Triceps-Biceps

By adding a second day to your MFT, you will accomplish more work. Rather than working all six major muscle groups in one day (chest, back, shoulders, legs, biceps, triceps), you will break down your workouts and focus on three different muscle groups for each workout. This is more common known as a "Split Routine." There are two different ways to determine which muscle groups you should be using in the same workout. The first is the agonist-antagonist method which explains that whenever you contract a muscle "agonist" there is an opposing muscle group that must relax "antagonist." Therefore, when choosing an exercise that works a joint in one direction, you should also select another exercise that works the joint in the opposite direction. For example, after working the chest muscles, you should work the back muscles. After working the bicep muscle, you should work the tricep muscle. The second way to choose what exercises to work on is to pair a large muscle group with a related smaller muscle group. For example, when you are working your chest, you are also working your triceps and when you are working your back, you are also working your biceps. Therefore, it makes sense to group the chest with the triceps and the back with the biceps during a workout. This way, you do not overwork the same muscle groups.

So, if you want to use the agonist/antagonist method than on Day 1 you should work the back and chest and then finish with the shoulders. Then give yourself at least 3 days off to recuperate the related smaller muscle groups (biceps and triceps). On Day 2, you will work the biceps and triceps, but remember that you do not have to perform as many sets of total work as you did with the larger muscle groups because the biceps and triceps are smaller and they will fatigue sooner and thus do not need as much work to overload them.

Table 7.4
Training for Muscular Fitness Three Days Per Week

	Week 1	Week 2	Week 3	Week 4
F	3	3	3	3
I	70%-90% of max or 2-8 reps per set	70%-90% of max or 2-8 reps per set	70%-90% of max or 2-8 reps per set	70%-90% of max or 2-8 reps per set
T	*Beginners* 2-3 exercises per body part; 1-2 sets per exercise; *Intermediate* 3 exercises per body part; 2-3 sets per exercise; *Advanced* 4 exercises per body part; 3 sets per exercise;	*Beginners* 2-3 exercises per body part; 2 sets per exercise; *Intermediate* 3-4 exercises per body part; 2-3 sets per exercise; *Advanced* 4-5 exercises per body part; 3-4 sets per exercise;	*Beginners* 3 exercises per body part; 2 sets per exercise; *Intermediate* 4 exercises per body part; 3 sets per exercise; *Advanced* 5 exercises per body part; 4 sets per exercise;	*Beginners* 3-4 exercises per body part 2-3 sets per exercise; *Intermediate* 4-5 exercises per body part; 3 sets per exercise; *Advanced* 5 exercises per body part; 4-5 sets per exercise;
T	Chest-Triceps Back Biceps Shoulders-Legs	Chest-Triceps Back-Biceps Shoulders-Legs	Chest-Back Shoulders-Legs Triceps-Biceps	Chest-Back Shoulders-Legs Triceps-Biceps

Table 7.5
Training for Muscular Fitness Four Days Per Week

	Week 1	Week 2	Week 3	Week 4
F	4	4	4	4
I	70%-90% of max or 2-8 reps per set	70%-90% of max or 2-8 reps per set	70%-90% of max or 2-8 reps per set	70%-90% of max or 2-8 reps per set
T	*Beginners* 2-3 exercises per body part; 1-2 sets per exercise on double muscle days; 2-3 exercises per body part; 2 sets per exercise on single muscle days; *Intermediate* 3 exercises per body part; 2 sets per exercise on single muscle days; 4 exercises per body part; 2 sets per exercise on single muscle days; *Advanced* 4 exercises per body part; 3 sets per exercise on double muscle days; 4-5 exercises per body part; 3-4 sets per exercise on single muscle days;	*Beginners* 3 exercises per body part; 2 sets per exercise on double muscle days; 3 exercises per body part; 2 sets per exercise on single muscle days; *Intermediate* 4 exercises per body part; 2 sets per exercise on double muscle days; 4 exercises per body part; 2-3 sets per exercise on single muscle days; *Advanced* 4-5 exercises per body part; 3-4 sets per exercise on double muscle days; 5 exercises per body part; 3-4 sets per exercise on single muscle days;	*Beginners* 3-4 exercises per body part; 2 sets per exercise on double muscle days; 4 exercises per body part; 2 sets per exercise on single muscle days; *Intermediate* 4 exercises per body part; 3 sets per exercise on double muscle days; 4-5 exercises per body part; 3 sets per exercise on single muscle days; *Advanced* 5 exercises per body part; 4 sets per exercise on double muscle days; 5-6 exercises per body part; 4 sets per exercise on single muscle days;	*Beginners* 3-4 exercises per body part 2-3 sets per exercise on double muscle days; 4 exercises per body part; 2-3 sets per exercise on single muscle days; *Intermediate* 4-5 exercises per body part; 3 sets per exercise on double muscle days; 5 exercises per body part; 3 sets per exercise on single muscle days; *Advanced* 5 exercises per body part; 4-5 sets per exercise on double muscle days; 5-6 exercises per body part; 4-5 sets per exercise on single muscle days;
T	Chest-Triceps Shoulders Back-Biceps Legs	Chest-Back Shoulder-Legs Biceps-Triceps	Chest Back Shoulders-Legs Triceps-Biceps	Chest-Triceps Back-Biceps Legs Shoulders

If you want to work the large and small related muscle groups always remember to work the large before the small. By working the large muscle group first, you are also working the related small. However, if you work the small muscle group first, it will fatigue sooner and not be able to help out the related large muscle group. For example on Day 1, you can work chest first followed by triceps and finish with shoulders. On Day 2, you can work back first followed by biceps and then finish with legs.

By adding a third day to your MFT, you will concentrate on working two body parts each workout day. Once again, by adding an extra day, you will accomplish more work on each body part.

Muscular Fitness Training Four Days Per Week

If you choose to work on your MF four days per week, you will begin to work one or two body parts per workout. If you are not working your chest and triceps or back and biceps on the same day, make sure you give yourself about 72 hours to recuperate from the large muscle group (chest and back) before working the related small muscle group (triceps and biceps). One advantage of training more times per week is if you are pressed for time on a given day, your workouts can be completed in a shorter time span because you are working less body parts. Moreover, you may be able to accomplish more work on a given body part.

It is important to note that smaller muscle groups (biceps and triceps) need less work than larger muscle groups (chest, back, shoulders). Therefore, when working a smaller muscle group by itself in a single workout, you should reduce the number of total sets of work by a few. This will decrease soreness and help the small muscle group to recuperate faster and be ready for the related larger muscle group workout.

Muscular Fitness Training Five Days Per Week

If you decide to work five days per week on your MF, you will be performing a one-body part workout on four of those days and a two-body part workout on one day. Rather than include a separate five-day per week schedule, you can follow the single muscle group workouts listed in the four-day per week program for four days and pair two body parts on the fifth day. Table 7.6 displays an example of how you can organize the body parts to work on in a five-day program.

Determining Your Level of Commitment to Muscular Fitness Training

As you learned in the previous chapter, your level of commitment, more than your actual fitness level, will determine how much, how often and how hard you will exercise. For some reason, one of the hardest parts of an exercise program seems to be scheduling the actual day(s) and time(s) to do your workout. Therefore, it is important for you to determine how many days per week you will commit to MFT. In addition, you should also identify what

Table 7.6
Training for Muscular Fitness Five Days Per Week

	Week 1	Week 2	Week 3	Week 4
F	5	5	5	5
I	70%-90% of max or 2-8 reps per set	70%-90% of max or 2-8 reps per set	70%-90% of max or 2-8 reps per set	70%-90% of max or 2-8 reps per set
T	*Beginners* 3 exercises per body part; 1-2 sets per exercise; *Intermediate* 3 exercises per body part; 2 sets per exercise; *Advanced* 4-5 exercises per body part; 3-4 sets per exercise;	*Beginners* 3-4 exercises per body part; 2 sets per exercise; *Intermediate* 3-4 exercises per body part; 3 sets per exercise; *Advanced* 4 exercises per body part; 4 sets per exercise;	*Beginners* 4 exercises per body part; 2 sets per exercise; *Intermediate* 4 exercises per body part; 3 sets per exercise; *Advanced* 4-5 exercises per body part; 4-5 sets per exercise;	*Beginners* 4-5 exercises per body part 2-3 sets per exercise; *Intermediate* 4-5 exercises per body part; 3-4 sets per exercise; *Advanced* 5 exercises per body part; 5 sets per exercise;
T	Chest Back Shoulders Legs Triceps-Biceps	Chest-Back Shoulders Legs Biceps Triceps	Legs Chest Back-Biceps Shoulders Triceps	Legs Back Chest-Triceps Shoulders Biceps

your goals are. Do you want to work on muscular strength and build your muscles? Do you want to shape, tone and define your muscles? Do you want a combination of both? In the previous section, you were introduced to three different MF programs designed to improve muscular strength, muscular endurance, or a combination of the two. Each program was also based on the number of days per week that you are committed toward working on MF.

So where are you on the commitment scale?

1	2	3	4	5	6	7	8	9
Low commitment			**Moderate Commitment**				**High Commitment**	

How many days per week will you commit to working on MF? 1 2 3 4 5

Based upon your level of commitment, you should consider one of the four-week MF programs presented above. Simply select the program that you have the highest level of commitment to follow over the next four weeks. Most important, enjoy yourself and have fun toning and strengthening your muscles.

SPICING UP YOUR PROGRAM

After a few weeks, your mind and body may begin to get used to the same old routine. Physically, you are not challenging your body as much because your muscles have become used to the same exercise in the same order during the same part of the week. Psychologically, you may become bored doing the same routine and not want to push yourself to get the extra rep or add a new exercise to your routine. To get the spice back into your program, you should consider making a few changes. Here are several ways you can do that:

1. ***Pyramids***—Increase the weight from one set to the next resulting in fewer reps performed from set to set. Although this tends to be a popular way of training, it is recommended to be used as a means to spice up your program rather than as your usual way of training since performing pyramids on every set of every exercise makes it difficult to overload properly. You are strongest on the first set, so raising the weight in later sets often results in individuals under-working themselves in the earlier sets just so they can conserve most of their energy to work harder in the later sets. Logically, if you are strongest in the earlier part of your workout and you want to improve, then you must overload your muscles at the beginning and work hard throughout the workout. That means lifting as much weight as you possibly can for the desired number of reps (e.g., 2-8, 8-12, 12-15) on all sets. It may be tempting to stop after a certain number of reps per set, even when you feel you can do more, so that you can "save your strength" for later sets. But in order to get the most out of your MF program, you should be overloading on eat set and lifting as much weight as you can for the desired number of reps. Pyramids are an excellent way to spice up your workout from time to time, but using pyramids should not become a regular part of your workout routine. Figure 7.5 demonstrates how to incorporate a pyramid correctly and incorrectly.

Body Part = Chest	Correct Pyramid	Incorrect Pyramid
Bench Press	100 lbs 12×	100 lbs 10×
	110 lbs 9×	120 lbs 8×
	115 lbs 6×	140 lbs 5×
	120 lbs 4×	160 lbs 3×
	125 lbs 2×	175 lbs 2×

Figure 7.5—Correct and Incorrect Ways to Use a Pyramid

As you can see in the correct pyramid, each time the weight was slightly increased, the number of reps went down. In other words, the workload from set to set was getting harder. In the incorrect pyramid, the weight is being substantially increased, yet the reps are only decreasing slightly. Moreover, if someone can lift 160 lbs in their 4th set, they most certainly could have done more than 10 reps of 100 lbs in the 1st set.

2. ***Super sets***—Consecutive exercise either of the same body area or a related body area performed without rest. For example, let's say you are working your chest and back and you plan to do two exercises from each body part. You can combine chest exercise 1 and 2 and then rest or you can do a chest exercise followed by a back exercise and then rest. By decreasing the rest time, you create a more intense overload. On the positive side, this will result in getting more fit. On the negative side, fatigue will set in faster during your workout which can create some difficulty working at the same rate of productivity forcing you to decrease weight and reps in the later sets.

Begin by warming up with an aerobic exercise for 1-2 minutes	Desired number of reps	Thoughts and feelings about how hard you are working; Amount of weight being used;
Bench Press	20-30 reps	
Lat Pulldown	20-30 reps	
Rhythmic Exercise	1-2 minutes	
Shoulder Press	20-30 reps	
Tricep Extension	20-30 reps	
Rhythmic Exercise	1-2 minutes	
Seated Row	20-30 reps	
Leg Press	20-25 reps	
Rhythmic Exercise	1-2 minutes	
Modified Front Raises	20-30 reps	Each time you raise your arm up, raise the same leg up
Pump N Walk	1-2 minutes	Each time you take a step walking, perform a bicep curl with the opposite arm; Make sure to use light weight.
Push ups	1 minute	
Curl Ups	1 minute	
Rhythmic Exercise	1-2 minutes	
	14-20 minutes	For intermediate or advanced fitness levels, you can either add more exercises or repeat the above-listed exercises. Intermediate Level – 30-45 minutes recommended Advanced Level – 30-60 minutes is recommended For those interested in working more on rhythmic exercises, you can alternate one rhythmic exercise for one resistance training exercise.

Figure 7.6—Circuit Training Workout

3. ***Circuit Training***—Combines muscular fitness with cardiorespiratory endurance in the same workout. First, select 8-12 resistance training exercises that incorporate all of the major muscle groups. Then you use approximately 40 to 50 percent of your max or select a weight that you can perform about 20-30 reps. Perform one set of two different resistance training exercise(s) and then perform a rhythmic exercise for 1-2 minutes that will get your heart rate up (e.g., jogging in place; stationary bicycle, shadow boxing, dancing, jump rope etc). Repeat cycle 4-8×. While circuit training is a creative way to exercise multiple systems (MF and CRE) and spice up your program, it does not work as efficiently as addressing each system separately for longer amount of time. See Figure 7.6 to see a circuit-training workout.

Incorporating the POC into your MF Program

To make sure your muscular fitness program is going to produce your desired results, you should make sure that you are incorporating each of the principles of conditioning into your program.

Warm Up Principle—An effective way to warm up before beginning to work on your muscular fitness is to select the exercise that you plan on doing in your workout and use a light weight or low intensity. This will let your body know how you will be working it and your mind know what you should be concentrating on. For example, say you performed 12-10-8 reps of 80 lbs on the bench press last week. Prior to performing your first set of bench press this week, you warm up with 40 lbs and do it 8-12 times. If you work out with very light weight, you can warm up by performing that exercise with no weight for 8-12 reps. See Figure 7.5 to see how to warm up with no weights.

Principle of Progression (POP)—The simplest way to incorporate the POP is to plan on increasing reps first followed by increasing the number of sets, then exercises and then adding weight. As you begin your MF program you will begin to see increases in muscular strength and endurance. Challenging yourself to do one more rep than last week, adding an exercise or doing an additional set will give you a sense of progress and keep you on the road to getting stronger, toning up and feeling great.

Principle of Individuality—Determine the number of days you work on MFT, the exercises you do, the weight you lift, and the sets and reps you prescribe for yourself based on your needs and not someone else's. The only way to do this is to use the information from your assessment to determine what your level of MF is and how many days you are willing to work out. Then follow the program that works for you.

Principle of Recuperation—Since MFT is a bit more intense on the muscles that CRE, you should make sure to provide adequate rest (at least 72 hours) after your muscles have been worked on before you plan to overload them again. Working each major muscle group once per week will give you sufficient rest time to recuperate from your workout overload and get you back at 100% for next week. When working the large muscle group with the related small muscle group in the same workout (e.g., chest with triceps; back with biceps) you are giving each body part six days of rest before being worked on again. When using the agonist-antagonist method (e.g., chest with back; triceps with biceps), you should work the larger muscle groups earlier in the week and give yourself at least 72 hours before working on the related small muscle groups). For example, if you plan on working out three times this week, you can start off working chest with back on Monday, shoulders with legs on Wednesday and triceps with biceps on Friday.

Principle of Fun—You can make your MF program fun in the identical way you are making your CRE program fun. Identify what you like that you can incorporate into your MF program: (music, exercise partner, finding the down time in the exercise facility so you can exercise alone; join a weight training class so you can work out with others).

Principle of Reversibility—In order to avoid losing what you have gained from over loading, you must work each of the major muscle groups once per week. If you are accustomed to working on your MF several times per week and your schedule suddenly changes and you only have one or two days, all you have to do is make sure you do a little of each of the six major muscle groups each week. This way you will be able to maintain your present level of MF until you get back to your usual routine.

Using SMAART Goals to Increase Muscular Fitness Motivation and Performance

To use SMAART goals to increase your MF all you need is your baseline MF level. Simply take the results of what you maxed on or the present level of weight that you are lifting and set any of the following goals: (1) increase max; (2) increase amount of weight being used during workouts; (3) increase exercises being performed each week; (4) increase

	Howie's SMAART Goals	My SMAART Goals
SPECIFIC	Improve Muscular Fitness & Get Stronger	
MEASURABLE	Be able to Max 150 lbs on the Bench Press	
ACTION-ORIENTED	Lift weights 3× per week and increase 2 sets per week over the next four weeks	
ADJUSTABLE	If Howie does not improve each week in either reps, sets or weight lifted, he will add a fourth day to his workouts or add a new exercise to make sure he increases his workout repetitions.	
REALISTIC	Howie maxed 130 lbs and by sticking to his program, he will be able to max 150 lbs in the near future.	
TIME-FRAME	Howie would like to reach his goal four weeks after he starts his MF program.	

Figure 7.7—Using SMAART Goals to Increase Muscular Fitness

sets and reps being performed each week or (5) increase the number of days working on MF; For example, let's say that you maxed 100 lbs on the leg press in week 1. You can set a goal to increase your max to 120 lbs by week 5. Perhaps you are lifting 6 sets per body part. Maybe you want to set a goal to achieve 7 sets by next week. Whatever motivates you the most to work hard on your MF is the goal(s) for you. Figure 7.7 includes an example of Howie, a man who wants to improve his muscular fitness and get stronger. He sets a measurable goal to be able to max 150 lbs on the bench press. He creates an action plan to lift

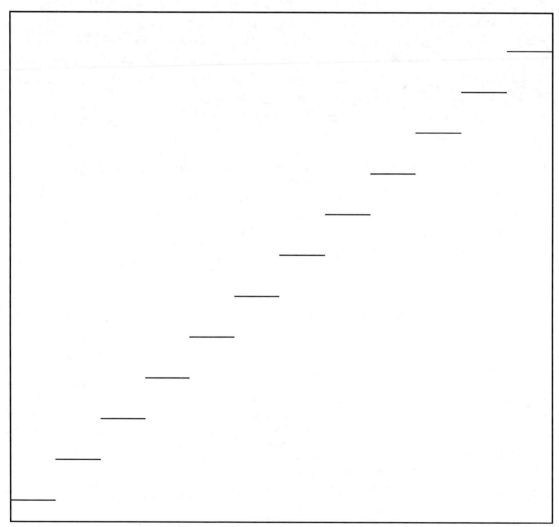

12-24 Week Stairway to Success...Put your baseline performance on the bottom of the stairs and today's date underneath. On the top of the stairs, write your long-term muscular fitness goal (what you would like to achieve in 6 months) and the date 6 months from now underneath that. On the stair next to your baseline, write your first short-term goal and the target date you are striving to reach it by. Each time you reach your short-term goal, you should set another goal on the next highest step along with your target date.

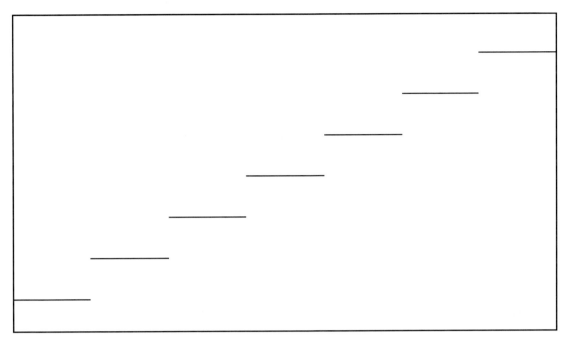

6-12 week Stairway to Success—This staircase can be used for goals that are desired to be reached over a 6-12 week period. Simply follow the guidelines for using the staircase outlined in the above 12-24 week stairway to success. The only difference is the top of your staircase is 6-12 weeks away from your bottom step baseline and each step represents one or two week short-term goal target dates.

Figure 7.8—Using the Stairway to Success to Set Short-Term and Long-Term Goals for MF

weights 3× per week and increase his total number of sets performed by two each week over a four-week period. If he does not improve each week, he will change his program around by increasing his frequency to a fourth day or adding exercises which will increase workout repetitions on the days that he works on his muscular fitness. The goal is realistic since Howie maxed 130 lbs before he began his muscular fitness program. Finally, Howie's time frame to reach his goal is four weeks from when he started which will certainly call him into action immediately. Figure 7.7 includes a blank column in the far right that is for you to fill in your SMAART goals to becoming more muscularly fit.

In addition to setting SMAART goals, if you have MF goals that you think may take longer than a few weeks to achieve, you can use Stairway to Success to set both short and long-term goals. For example, let's say you are up to six sets of work in week 1 and you would like to be able to achieve 25 sets in a given workout. Using the Stairway, you can map out your baseline of 6 sets on the bottom of the steps and your long-term goal of 25 sets on the top. Then use each step starting with the step above the baseline as a short-term goal. Each time you reach your short-term goal, simply move up one step until you get to the top of the stairs. See Figure 7.8 to set Staircase goals to improve your level of MF.

EVALUATING THE SUCCESS OF YOUR MUSCULAR FITNESS PROGRAM

Have you followed your exercise prescription? Are you as committed as you thought you would be? Do you see improvements from Week 1 to Week 4 in the amount of weight lifted, reps and sets achieved, number of exercises being performed? Do you feel better after a workout? Has your recuperation time decreased? Does soreness or discomfort subside quicker? Do you look forward to working on MF? Has your body improved in muscular size? definition? tone? firmness? Did you reach your goals? These are all ways for you to evaluate the success of your program? If you answered "NO" to any of these questions then you should determine what is stopping you and develop a plan of action to overcome these barriers and get back on track.

Preventing Injuries

There are several strategies that you can incorporate to reduce injuries and they include:

Warming up—Prior to overloading your muscles you should warm up by performing 8-12 reps of a light weight with the exercises you plan on using in your workout;

Learning proper form of exercises—Before selecting an exercise, make sure you know how to do it properly. If you are taking a class, the instructor should demonstrate how to do it. If you belong to a gym, ask the manager or personal trainer to show you how. Take the text book with you and model the pictures labeled "correct form." Finally, using either no or very little weight, practice your exercises a few times and concentrate on proper seating or standing position, incorporating the proper range of motion and going slowly.

Spotting—Use of a partner to assist you in your workout. The spotter's primary responsibility is safety: knowing the correct form of the exercise being performed, the ability of the individual lifting (e.g., how many reps he/she is planning on doing), proper breathing techniques and the proper positioning for the exercise being performed (e.g., range of motion, incline, decline, upright, lying on back, lying on stomach). The spotter is not there to help the individual lift the weight, only to make sure that the individual is lifting the weight safely.

Breathing Properly—You should exhale on the exertion phase (lifting the weight) and inhale on the resting phase (when the weight returns to its starting position). The exertion phase takes 1-2 seconds while the resting phase should take 3-4 seconds. That means each rep should take 4-6 seconds to complete.

Know your exercise—Some exercises can cause injury if done improperly and they include: (1) arching your back when laying flat (e.g., bench press); (2) locking your knees during a leg press or leg extension; (3) putting the handle bar behind your neck on the lat pull down; Therefore, know the exercise before planning to use it in your MF program.

In this chapter you have learned the benefits of participating in a muscular fitness program. You have been introduced to two different methods of assessing your MF as well as a variety of different MF programs to choose from. You should be able to find at least one program that you are highly committed to using so that you can improve your MF. Please proceed onto the review questions and lab assignment for Chapter 7 so you can test your knowledge and continue to develop your expertise.

REVIEW QUESTIONS

1. Describe a common myth associated with women who participate in weight training and explain how you would disprove this myth to a bunch of believers.

2. Define the two components of muscular fitness?

3. List five or more benefits of being muscularly fit. Which of these benefits increases your motivation to start or continue working on your muscular fitness?

4. List and explain a procedure for assessing muscular strength.

5. List and explain a procedure for assessing muscular endurance.

6. How would you measure the four components of an exercise prescription for muscular fitness?

7. Explain the difference in intensity being used for someone who wants to tone/define his/her muscles and someone who wants to increase muscular size.

8. What five questions would you ask someone in order to determine proper time involved in a muscular fitness program?

9. What are the main differences between someone who is training on muscular fitness one day per week and someone else who is training four days per week?

10. Describe two strategies you would consider to spice up your muscular fitness program.

11. Explain the correct and incorrect ways of using a pyramid to work on muscular fitness.

12. Discuss how you plan to use goal setting to improve your muscular fitness and create a high level of motivation to continue over the next 3-6 months.

13. What can you do to prevent injuries while working on your muscular fitness?

Lab Assignment 7.1

Questions 1-9 should be answered prior to beginning your MF fitness program.

1. How committed are you to improving your MF fitness over the next four weeks? If you have a low level of commitment, what strategies will you incorporate to increase your level of commitment?

2. What are your SMAART goals for improving your MF over the next 4 weeks?

   A. _____

   B. _____

   C. _____

3. Using the stairway to success, convert your SMAART goals into stairway goals set your goals over the next four weeks.

   _____

                              _____

              _____

       _____

4. Develop an exercise prescription to improve your MF fitness over the next four weeks.

	Week 1	Week 2	Week 3	Week 4
F				
I				
T				
T				

5. Explain how you plan to comply with the principle of progression over the next four weeks.

6. Describe how you plan to incorporate the principle of recuperation into your MF program?

7. How will you incorporate the principle of warm up into your MF program?

8. What strategies are you considering to incorporate the principle of fun into your MF program?

9. What strategies do you have planned to avoid the principle of reversibility?

Questions 10-14 should be answered at the conclusion of each week.

10. Explain how you have been overloading from weeks' 1-2-3-4?

11. How has your recuperation time changed from weeks' 1-4?

12. How successful were you in avoiding the principle of reversibility?

13. Using the chart located in Appendix 6A, discuss how much have your improved from weeks' 1-4?

14. Did you have fun while working on your MF fitness? If so, explain the strategies that you have incorporated to have fun? If you did not have fun, explain what you plan to do over the next few weeks to make your MF workouts more fun (e.g., music, exercising with a partner, etc).

REFERENCES AND RECOMMENDED READINGS

American College of Sports Medicine (2002). Position Stand: Progression Models in Resistance Training for Healthy Adults. Medicine and Science in Sport and Exercise, 34(2), 364-380.

Brzycki, M. (1999). "Free weights and machines." *Fitness Management, 15*, 36-37 40.

Hakkinen, K. (2004). Changes in muscle hypertrophy in women with periodized resistance training. *Medicine and Science in Sports and Exercise, 36, 4,* 697-708.

Hesson, J. (2007). Weight training for life, 8th addition. Wadsworth/Thomson Learning.

Hoeger, W. WK., Hopkins, D.R., Barette, S.L., & Hale, D.F. (1990). Relationship between repetitions and selected percentages of one repetition maximum: A comparison between untrained and trained males and females. *Journal of Applied Sport Science Research, 4,* 47-51.

Kraemer, W.J., & Ratamess, N.A. (2004). Fundamentals of resistance training: Progression and exercise prescriptions. *Medicine and Science in Sports and Exercise, 36, 4,* 674-689.

Powers, S.K., & Howley, E.T. (2004). Exercise physiology: Theory and application to fitness and performance. 5th edition. McGraw-Hill.

Rhea, M.R., Alvar, B.A., Ball, S.D., & Burkett, L.N. (2002). Three sets of weight training superior to 1 set with equal intensity for eliciting strength. *Journal of Strength Conditioning Research, 16*, 525-529.

Smith, D., & Bruce-Low, S. (2004). Strength training methods and the work of Arthur Jones .*Journal of Exercise Physiology, 7, 6,* 52-62.

www.acsm-msse.org.

APPENDIX 7A
HOW MUCH HAVE YOU IMPROVED OVER THE LAST FOUR WEEKS

	Week 1	Week 2	Week 3	Week 4
Days Exercised				
Body Parts Addressed				
Exercises Selected				
Sets Achieved				
Reps Achieved				

1. Discuss how you feel about your improvements over the last four weeks?

2. My motivation to continue working on muscular fitness has

        decreased   remained the same   increased

3. If your motivation has decreased or remained the same, explain why and then list your strategies to increase your motivation over the next one to four weeks.

4. If you motivation has increased, use Appendix 7B to develop your action plan over the next four weeks.

5. What goals will you strive to reach over the next week? Use Appendix 7C to set your weekly muscular fitness goals.

APPENDIX 7B
ACTION PLAN FOR DEVELOPING OR IMPROVING MUSCULAR FITNESS

	Week 1	Week 2	Week 3	Week 4
The actions I will take over the next four weeks to reach my muscular fitness goals are:				
Action 1				
Action 2				
Action 3				
Action 4				
Action 5				

APPENDIX 7C
WEEKLY GOAL SHEET FOR CRE

Name _____ Date: _____

Select 1-2 goals that will help you improve your Muscular Fitness this week. Write down your goal(s) in the "Goal(s) Selected" column next to the category of goal that you have selected. Using the 7 Day Chart down below, record each day's workout next to the appropriate activity and under the actual day. After the week is up, add up your total workout performances and put them in the "Performance Results" column. If you achieved you weekly goal, mark an "A" across from your goal category in the "Achieved" column. If you did not reach your goal, mark an "NA" across from you goal category and under the "Not Achieved" column.

Muscular Fitness Goals to Select From	Goal(s) Selected	Performance Results	Achieved = A	Not Achieved = NA
Frequency of Weekly Muscular Fitness Workouts				
Number of Exercises Completed for Week				
Number of Sets Completed for Week				
Number of Reps Completed for Week				
Exercises Increasing in Weight				

Muscular Fitness	Day 1	Day 2	Day 3	Day 4	Day 5	Day 6	Day 7
Exercises Completed							
Sets Completed							
Reps Completed							
Exercises Increasing in Weight							

Chapter 8
Developing an Exercise Prescription for Flexibility

OBJECTIVES

After this chapter, you will be able to:

- Understand the benefits and importance of being flexible
- Formally and informally assess your flexibility
- Develop an exercise prescription for improving your flexibility
- Determine your level of commitment to being more flexible
- Set S-M-A-A-R-T goals to improve and enjoy your flexibility program
- Learn how to minimize and prevent injuries while engaging in flexibility exercises

Flexibility is the least worked on component of health-related fitness. Some people do not know how to stretch properly while others do not recognize the importance of being flexible. Today much research has been done on the importance of being flexible as well as how to stretch properly (Alter, 1996; Liemohn, 2003;). Unfortunately, knowledge by itself is not enough to get people motivated to work on improving their flexibility. Factors such as boredom, not seeing results, being inconvenienced, misinterpreting tension for pain and to a lesser extent not knowing exactly what to do have all been recognized as barriers that stop individuals from being motivated to improve their flexibility. By the end of this chapter, you will be motivated to "stretch out your schedule" and fit flexibility into your daily routine.

WHAT IS MUSCULAR FLEXIBILITY?

Flexibility is defined as the ability of a joint to move through its full range of motion. Being flexible means feeling "loose" and being able to move your body around freely and comfortably without pain. However, being flexible in one part of the body does not mean that you are equally as flexible in another. For example, you can be very loose in your upper body and have full range of motion in your arms, shoulders and chest and have a limited range of motion in your legs and have difficulty touching your toes.

137

As you get older, your flexibility naturally decreases which increases your chances of aches, pains, and injuries. The only solution is to be "flexible" and make the commitment to find the time to work on increasing your range of motion.

Benefits of Flexibility

There are many benefits to being more flexible and they include:
1. increased ability to move around freely
2. reduced injury frequency and severity
3. increased motor performance
4. increased joint mobility
5. improved body position and strength needed for sport performance
6. improved posture
7. decreased muscle soreness
8. fewer aches and pains
9. fewer low back problems
10. reduction of stress

Assessing Your Flexibility

As you learned in Chapter 6, there are both formal and informal ways to assess health-related fitness. While both cardiorespiratory endurance and muscular strength may be assessed in a variety of ways (e.g., 1.5 mile run, step test, 12 minute swim, max testing, sub max test), flexibility assessments are limited due to lack of joint specific equipment. Presently, there are only a handful of formal assessments, none of which measure flexibility in all parts of the body. Therefore, in order to determine one's true level of flexibility, a combination of formal and informal assessments should be considered in order to gain more accurate information on how flexible you are in all areas of the body rather than in one or two places.

---

1. Warm up first by moving around continuously for a few minutes (e.g., walking briskly, light jogging, stationary bicycle).
2. Take your shoes off. Sit on the floor with your head, shoulders, and back against a wall.
3. Fully extend your legs so that your heels are up against the sit & reach box.
4. Keep your knees locked.
5. Place one hand on top of the other and move the lever as far forward as possible. Repeat twice for a total of three trials.
6. Record your highest number in either inches or centimeters to the nearest half.

Formal and Informal Assessments

The two most common formal assessments for flexibility are the sit and reach and the trunk rotation tests. See Figures 8.1 and 8.2 for procedures on how to perform each assessment.

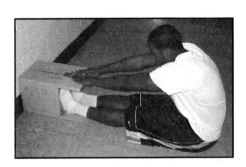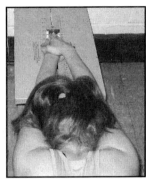

Figure 8.1—Procedures for Performing Sit and Reach Test

1. Tape two yardsticks to the wall at shoulder height, one right side up and the other upside down. The numbers should read 1-36 right side up on the left side and 1-36 upside down on the right side.
2. Stand with your left shoulder arm's distance from the wall. Toes should be facing straight ahead, perpendicular to the wall and even with the 15-inch mark of the left yardstick.
3. Drop the left arm and raise the right arm to the side.
4. Without moving your feet, rotate your trunk to the right as far as possible as you reach along the yardstick.
5. Hold for 3-4 seconds and do not move your feet or bend the trunk. You can bend your knees slightly.
6. Have a partner record the distance reached to the nearest half-inch. Repeat two times and record your highest score.
7. Change directions with your right should arm's distance from the wall. This time you will rotate to the left and use the second yardstick (the one that is upside down).

Figure 8.2—Procedures for Performing Trunk Rotation Test

While these assessments provide valuable information about how flexible you are in these specific areas, they do not tell you how flexible you are throughout the rest of your body. So in order to design an individualized flexibility program, you will need to conduct a series of informal assessments using a variety of commonly used flexibility exercises. Your goal is to stretch all of your major muscle groups and measure two criteria: (1) your tension point and (2) how long you can hold your stretch at your tension point. Your tension point is the furthest spot you can hold a stretch. For example, if you are doing a modified hurdler's stretch and the furthest you can reach is your ankles, then your tension point would be your ankles. Use Table 8.1 to informally assess your flexibility. By using a combination of standardized (formal) assessments with traditional flexibility exercises and measuring your tension point along with the amount of time you held each stretch, you will learn exactly how flexible you are throughout your body; with this knowledge, you can design a flexibility program that is just right for you.

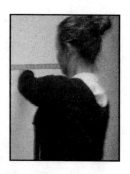

Table 8.1
Informally Assessing Your Flexibility

Flexibility Exercises	Area(s) Being Assessed	Tension Point Achieved	Length of Time Held	Level of Comfort	Level of Enjoyment
Lateral Head Tilt	Neck				
Head Turn	Neck				
Wrap Around	Shoulder & Neck				
Arm Lift	Chest & Shoulders				
Zipper	Shoulders, Arms & Chest				
Across the Body	Shoulders & Upper Back				
Trunk Rotation	Shoulders, Lower Back & Hips				
Towel Stretch	Chest, Shoulders, Triceps				
Triceps Stretch	Triceps & Shoulders				
Lateral Stretch	Trunk				
Sit & Reach	Hamstring & lower back				
Knee to Chest	Hip, Hamstrings & lower back				
Ankle Flex	Calf				
Back Extension	Abdominals				
Side Stretch	Pelvis,				
Quad Stretch	Quadriceps, Hip Flexors, Knees, Ankles				
Hip Flexor Stretch	Hip Flexors				
Sitting Adductor	Hip Adductors				
Modified Hurdler's Stretch	Hamstring, Lower Back				
Single Knee to Chest	Lower back & hamstrings				
Double Knee to Chest	Upper & lower back & hamstrings;				
Step Stretch	Hips, Quadriceps				
Push the Wall	Calf, hamstring				
Arm Across	Shoulders, Arms				
Toes to Step	Calf				

To determine your level of comfort/discomfort during your flexibility assessment, please answer the following question and place your answer in the column marked "level of comfort."

This exercise was

1	2	3	4	5	6	7
Very			Neither			Very
Comfortable						Uncomfortable

To determine your level of enjoyment performing each stretch, please answer the following question and place your answer in the column marked "level of enjoyment."

I enjoyed this flexibility exercise

1	2	3	4	5	6	7
Not at all						Very much

TYPES OF STRETCHING TECHNIQUES

There are several different stretching techniques you can use to improve your flexibility that range from safe to unsafe and simple to complex. These include:

Static Stretch (SS)—In this type of exercise, you stretch a muscle to a certain point where you feel tension and then hold it for a prescribed time period (e.g., 10-20 seconds). The *benefits* of static stretching are: (1) that it is easy to do; (2) it is the safest of all flexibility techniques; (3) you can do it by yourself and (4) you will certainly improve your flexibility. The *limitation* is that by yourself, you may not be able to reach your true tension point due to physical limitations. For example, when performing the modified hurdler's stretch by your-self you will get to a certain point and not be able to stretch any further. However, with some assistance from a partner, you are able to achieve a greater range of motion and stretch farther. See Figure 8.3 to compare the range of motion achieved with the static and passive static stretching techniques.

Ballistic Stretch—"Ballistic" refers to a bouncing motion: when you perform a ballistic stretch you are bouncing your muscles up and down or back and forth, repeatedly. To get a clear picture of a ballistic stretch, imagine your muscles being like a frozen rubber band. You take the rubber band out of the freezer and try to quickly stretch it back and forth. The end result would be a broken rubber band. That is exactly what could happen when you stretch ballistically. The *benefit* of stretching ballistically is that you can improve your level of flexibility as long as you bounce slowly, gently and in a controlled motion. The *limitation* is that ballistic stretching can be dangerous if bouncing is done in a rapid, jerky motion. This can cause overstretching which can lead to soreness and possible injury due to the tearing of soft tissue.

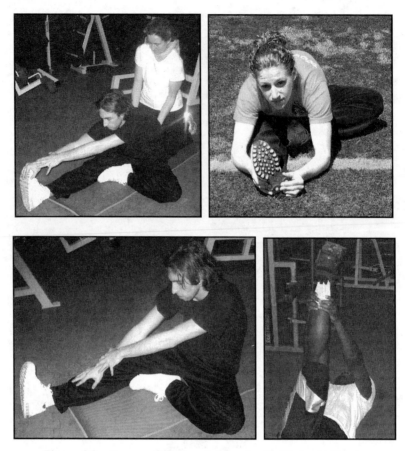

***Figure 8.3—Range of Motion Achieved with Static vs. Passive
Static Stretching Techniques***

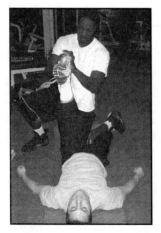

    Proprioceptive Neuromsucular Facilitation (PNF)—PNF
stretching involves the use of a partner to assist you in stretching.
It is based on a contract-relax sequence where your partner creates
some force by pushing you slowly in the direction of your desired
stretch. You then, apply force in the opposite direction against
your partner. Your partner will hold you in this position for 5-10
seconds, thus creating an isometric contraction (force is being
exerted without any movement). Then your partner will increase
the resistance by holding you at a greater angle. You repeat the
isometric contraction for another 5-10 seconds and then relax. The
process can be performed anywhere from 2-5 times for as little as
5 seconds or as long as 30 seconds. (See Figure 8.4 to view a PNF
stretch). The *benefits* of PNF stretching are that: (1) it creates a

better range of motion that static stretching because of the use of a partner to help you stretch and (2) it will improve muscular fitness due to the isometric contraction being performed for prescribed lengths of time (5-30 seconds). The *limitations* are that: (1) PNF stretching has been known to cause muscle stiffness and soreness; (2) PNF stretching takes more time to complete than static stretching and (3) PNF stretching requires a knowledgeable partner who knows how to perform the exercises correctly as well as understanding your present level of flexibility and therefore how much pressure to exert. In addition, individuals sometimes like to exercise alone and feel uncomfortable asking someone else for assistance?

Passive Static—Passive static stretching usually involves the use of a partner to help you stretch and achieve your full range of motion. The partner serves as an outside force to push you in the desired direction of the stretch. For example, you want to stretch your hamstrings and lower back and decide to do the sit and reach stretch. By yourself, you can reach as far as your ankles. Your partner now places some force in the center of your back and now you are able to reach your toes. Passive static stretching can also be performed by yourself, using objects like towels or light resistance bands to create an enhanced range of motion. For example, you can use a towel to assist you in a hamstring stretch. Simply lay flat on your back and put a towel around the ball of your foot and move the edges of the towel to your face. Holding the towel in this position enables you to move your leg closer to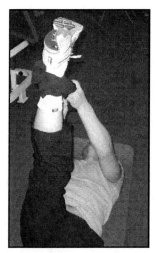
you and create a greater range of motion. (See Figure 8.5 to view a passive static towel stretch). The *benefit* of passive static stretching is that it will enable you to stretch to a further point than a static stretch. In addition, having a partner with you may also increase your motivation to stretch. The main *limitation* of passive static stretching is lack of communication. When working with a partner, the following information must be discussed: (1) the exercise(s) being performed; (2) how long the stretch is to be held for; (3) the desired tension point and (4) when the individual has had enough and needs to stop; The partner must know the proper form of all exercises being performed as well as the ability of the individual stretching. It is also important for the partner to listen to the individual and not force him/her to overstretch by going past the proper tension point or holding longer than can be comfortably withstood. Failure to do so can result in injury.

COMMON PROBLEMS AND SOLUTIONS ASSOCIATED WITH STRETCHING

For many years, flexibility was equated with warming up. Whether in physical education class, practice for sports or getting ready to go for your morning jog, traditionally, individuals would start out with a few stretches and then begin their activity. Although flexibility and warming up are related, they are not the same thing. Warming up means getting your body ready for action, usually through large muscle activity (e.g., brisk walk, light jog, stationary bicycle) for a few minutes prior to the start of your workout. It also means working the same muscles you plan to overload at a slower or lighter intensity motion (e.g., performing 8-12 reps with a light weight before increasing to a weight that will create overload), while stretching involves moving your joints through their full range of motion. To stretch before warming up is like trying to quench your thirst with a cup of ice cubes: the ice cubes will eventually melt, but it will take some time before they are converted into water and can be used as a drink to satisfy your thirst. Your muscles are cold and tight and really cannot be stretched effectively without being warmed up first. You may get a little looser, but it will hardly be an effective stretch, just as the ice cubes by themselves will hardly make an effective drink by themselves. Below are some common problems that occur when stretching, along with ways of preventing them.

Going too fast—Sometimes we view stretching as a prelude to another activity and so we rush through a few stretches by rapidly moving to a point where we feel tension, holding for a few seconds and then moving to the next activity. The problem is that we may never give ourselves enough time to elongate the muscle. *Solution:* Go slow. Stretch to a point where you feel tension and hold it for at least 10 seconds. Then try to stretch farther. The slower you go and the longer you can hold a stretch, the further you will be able to stretch and the better you will feel.

Not reaching tension point—It is tempting to stretch until you feel a little bit of tension and then stop. While doing so will improve your flexibility somewhat (provided you hold the stretch for at least 10 seconds), you are not stretching to your true tension point and thus not getting an effective stretch. That is like lifting 40 percent of your max and stopping after 10 reps. *Solution:* Stretch as far as you can and hold for at least 10 seconds. Every five seconds try to stretch a little further.

No pain no gain—Some people believe that in order to see results they must feel pain. That is simply not true: there is a fine line between tension and pain. Feeling tension while stretching means you are overloading the intended area, which results in improvement. Feeling pain while stretching often means overstretching or not using the proper technique. *Solution*: Learn where your tension point is and challenge yourself to reach it and not go past it. You should be experiencing a moderate amount of tension while stretching, and the longer you hold the stretch, the less tension you should feel. If you are experiencing pain then shorten the distance that you are stretching. Always avoid full flexion and extension of the knees and neck.

Holding your breath—Sometimes people hold their breath while stretching. This makes it difficult to stretch for prolonged periods of time or concentrate on stretching to the true tension point. *Solution:* Inhale before you start to feel tension and then slowly exhale once you begin to hold at your tension point. As you exhale, imagine the tension being evaporated from the bodily area being stretched. You can also count to yourself while inhaling and exhaling.

This will help you to stretch longer and make sure you are breathing properly and not holding your breath.

Not seeing results—Just as there is less equipment available for flexibility than for CRE and MF workouts, there is also less material (e.g., workout cards, progress sheets) to record your flexibility workouts. Thus, it is easy to forget what was done during a flexibility workout. This decreases one's level of motivation to continue and makes it difficult to set S-M-A-A-R-T goals. *Solution:* Record your results. Write down the exercises you do, the length of time for which you hold each stretch, your present tension point, your desired tension, and your flexibility goals. (See Appendix 8A for a log to record your flexibility workouts and see your progress.

Boredom—Holding a stretch for a certain length of time can become quite boring for some people especially when little if any movement is required and the focus is on the tension being felt. *Solution:* Find something you like to do while stretching. For example, play your favorite music or stretch with a partner and start up a friendly conversation. This will help you to associate stretching with what you like to do and thus increase your motivation to improve your flexibility. In Chapter 11, you will be introduced to cognitive strategies that teach you how and what to think during various modes of exercise (e.g., flexibility, CRE, MF).

DEVELOPING AN EXERCISE PRESCRIPTION FOR IMPROVING YOUR FLEXIBILITY

By now you should realize that working on flexibility is a very important part of your health-related fitness. Now it is time to develop your own exercise prescription for flexibility so that you can get started working in this area and feel good about what you are accomplishing. While the same four components of an exercise prescription are used (F-I-T-T), the way each is measured is slightly different for flexibility than CRE or MF.

Frequency—How many days will you commit to flexibility? While it is commonly recommended by fitness experts that you should work on flexibility at least 3-5 days per week, this may or may not be realistic for you especially if you are not presently active or if dislike working on flexibility. Therefore, you should decide how many days you will commit to working on flexibility and remember that stretching does not have to take as long as CRE or MFT to see and feel good results.

Intensity—the intensity of your flexibility program is defined and measured by your tension point. You tension point is the furthest point at which you can hold a stretch. For example, if the furthest spot you can reach to on the modified hurdler's stretch is your shins, then your tension point is your shins for that stretch.

Time—Time can be defined and measured in two ways: (1) the number of exercises you plan to do and (2) the number of seconds you plan to hold each stretch. For example,

Michelle has selected five stretches to work on and she plans to hold each stretch for 10-15 seconds each. Therefore, she will stretch for a total of 50-75 seconds.

Type—Type is also defined and measured in two ways: (1) the flexibility technique that you are using (e.g., static, passive static, PNF) and (2) the name of the stretches you select (e.g., quad stretch, groin stretch, towel stretch).

Of the four components of your exercise prescription, the one that is the most related to your level of commitment is "F." Once you have decided how many days per week you will commit to working on flexibility, the I, T, and T should be easy for you to follow. For "Type," you should select different stretches that work all of your major muscle groups from head to toe and decide what techniques work best to increase your range of motion (e.g., static, passive static, PNF). Below is a procedure for you to follow that will help you design your flexibility exercise prescription.

1. Using your Flexibility Exercise Prescription Form, circle the number of days that you are committing to work on flexibility in week 1 (See Figure 8.6).
2. Decide how many stretches you will do in Week 1 and the duration of each stretch for.
3. Select the flexibility exercises that you plan to do in week 1 and the technique(s) that you will use (e.g., static, passive static, PNF).
4. Warm up before stretching
5. Stretch slowly and gently

	Week 1	Week 2	Week 3	Week 4
F	1-2-3-4-5-6-7	1-2-3-4-5-6-7	1-2-3-4-5-6-7	1-2-3-4-5-6-7
I	Present Tension Point listed on Flexibility Workout Card	Desired Tension Point listed on Flexibility Workout Card	Desired Tension Point Listed on Flexibility Workout Card	Desired Tension Point Listed on Flexibility Workout Card
T—list the number of stretches you will do each week & how long you plan to hold each stretch for				
T—list the technique that you will us (SS, PS, PNF) & the names of the flexibility exercises that you will consider				

Figure 8.6—Flexibility Exercise Prescription Form

Flexibility Exercises		Wk 1 Day 1	Wk 1 Day 2	Wk 2 Day 3	Wk 2 Day 4	Wk 3 Day 5	Wk 3 Day 6	Wk 3 Day 7	Wk 4 Day 8	Wk 4 Day 9	Wk 4 Day 10
1. Sit / Reach Stretch	Sec Held / Sets / TP	10 / 1 / ankles	10 / 1 / ankles		Middle of foot			Base of toes			top of toes
2. Quad Stretch	Sec Held / Sets / TP	10 / 1 / heel 2 inches from buttocks	10 / 1 / heel 2 inches from buttocks		heel 1 inch from buttocks			heel touching buttocks	heel touching buttocks		
3. Knee to Chest	Sec Held / Sets / TP	10 / 1 / knee to abdomen	10 / 1 / knee to abdomen		knee to bottom of chest			knee to mid chest			knee to top of chest
4. Tricep Stretch	Sec Held / Sets / TP	10 / 1 / elbow to top of head	10 / 1 / elbow to top of head		elbow to ear			elbow to back of neck			elbow to back of neck
5. Hip Flexor Stretch	Sec Held / Sets / TP	10 / 1 / front knee over middle of foot			front knee over base of toes			front knee to bottom of toes			front knee over top of toes
6. Sitting Twist	Sec Held / Sets / TP				front shoulder to belly button			front shoulder to opposite pectoralis			front shoulder to opposite hip
7. Lateral Head Tilt *partner needed to measure TP	Sec Held / Sets / TP							head 3 inches from shoulder			head 2 inches from shoulder

Figure 8.7—Mindy's Flexibility Workout Card

6. Stretch to your tension point

7. Breath slowly and consistently

Once you have finished, you can record your results on your flexibility workout card located in Appendix 8A. Then you can use your results from week 1 (e.g., number of days you worked on flexibility, number of stretches completed, seconds held for each stretch, tension point achieved for each exercise) to design your Flexibility Exercise Prescription for weeks 2, 3, and 4. You see, once you have completed week 1, you can use your results to improve your flexibility by adding more stretches in the upcoming weeks, striving to hold each stretch a few seconds longer and reaching new tension points. Below is an example that demonstrates how to record your results and from week 1 and use it to progress in weeks' 2-4. Paula is a college freshman who worked on flexibility two times in Week 1. She performed stretches 1-5 on her Flexibility Workout Card (See Figure 8.7) and she held each stretch for 10 seconds. As a result of her performance in Week 1, Paula has designed the following flexibility exercise prescription for Weeks' 2-4 (See Figure 8.8).

As you can see, Paula has increased the length of time she stretched in Week 1 by holding each stretch for a longer time and adding exercises in Weeks' 2-4. In addition, Paula has identified where she would like her tension point to be in each of the seven exercises she plans to do. Because, she now strives to stretch further and longer each week, Paula will see a significant improvement in her flexibility over time. Now you should have a clear understanding of how to develop and implement your Flexibility Exercise Prescription and record your results. If Paula can do it, then so can you!

	WEEK 1	WEEK 2	WEEK 3	WEEK 4
F	1-**2**-3-4-5-6-7	1-**2**-3-4-5-6-7	1-**2**-**3**-4-5-6-7	1-**2**-**3**-4-5-6-7
I	Present Tension Point listed on Flexibility Workout Card	Desired Tension Point listed on Flexibility Workout Card	Desired Tension Point Listed on Flexibility Workout Card	Desired Tension Point Listed on Flexibility Workout Card
T	5 exercises held for 10 seconds each	5-6 exercises held for 12 seconds each	6 exercises held for 12-14 seconds each	6-7 exercises held for 15 seconds each
T	Sit & Reach (SS) Quad Stretch (SS) Knee to Chest (SS) Tricep Stretch (SS) Hip Flexor Stretch (SS)	Sit & Reach (PS) Quad Stretch (SS) Knee to Chest (SS) Tricep Stretch (SS) Hip Flexor Stretch (SS) Lateral Head Tilt (SS)	Sit & Reach (PS) Quad Stretch (SS) Knee to Chest (PNF) Tricep Stretch (SS) Hip Flexor Stretch (SS) Lateral Head Tilt (SS)	Sit & Reach (PS) Quad Stretch (SS) Knee to Chest (PNF) Tricep Stretch (SS) Hip Flexor Stretch (SS) Lateral Head Tilt (SS) Wrap Around (SS)

SS—static stretch; PS—passive static stretch; PNF—proprioceptive neuromuscular facilitation stretch

Figure 8.8—Paula's Flexibility Exercise Prescription

Time	Monday	Tuesday	Wednesday	Thursday	Friday	Saturday	Sunday
7-8 AM	3 4 5 6 7 8 9 10 11 12 13 14 15 16 17 18 19 20	3 4 5 6 7 8 9 10 11 12 13 14 15 16 17 18 19 20	3 4 5 6 7 8 9 10 11 12 13 14 15 16 17 18 19 20	3 4 5 6 7 8 9 10 11 12 13 14 15 16 17 18 19 20	3 4 5 6 7 8 9 10 11 12 13 14 15 16 17 18 19 20	3 4 5 6 7 8 9 10 11 12 13 14 15 16 17 18 19 20	3 4 5 6 7 8 9 10 11 12 13 14 15 16 17 18 19 20
8-9 AM	3 4 5 6 7 8 9 10 11 12 13 14 15 16 17 18 19 20	3 4 5 6 7 8 9 10 11 12 13 14 15 16 17 18 19 20	3 4 5 6 7 8 9 10 11 12 13 14 15 16 17 18 19 20	3 4 5 6 7 8 9 10 11 12 13 14 15 16 17 18 19 20	3 4 5 6 7 8 9 10 11 12 13 14 15 16 17 18 19 20	3 4 5 6 7 8 9 10 11 12 13 14 15 16 17 18 19 20	3 4 5 6 7 8 9 10 11 12 13 14 15 16 17 18 19 20
9-10 AM	3 4 5 6 7 8 9 10 11 12 13 14 15 16 17 18 19 20	3 4 5 6 7 8 9 10 11 12 13 14 15 16 17 18 19 20	3 4 5 6 7 8 9 10 11 12 13 14 15 16 17 18 19 20	3 4 5 6 7 8 9 10 11 12 13 14 15 16 17 18 19 20	3 4 5 6 7 8 9 10 11 12 13 14 15 16 17 18 19 20	3 4 5 6 7 8 9 10 11 12 13 14 15 16 17 18 19 20	3 4 5 6 7 8 9 10 11 12 13 14 15 16 17 18 19 20
10-11 AM	3 4 5 6 7 8 9 10 11 12 13 14 15 16 17 18 19 20	3 4 5 6 7 8 9 10 11 12 13 14 15 16 17 18 19 20	3 4 5 6 7 8 9 10 11 12 13 14 15 16 17 18 19 20	3 4 5 6 7 8 9 10 11 12 13 14 15 16 17 18 19 20	3 4 5 6 7 8 9 10 11 12 13 14 15 16 17 18 19 20	3 4 5 6 7 8 9 10 11 12 13 14 15 16 17 18 19 20	3 4 5 6 7 8 9 10 11 12 13 14 15 16 17 18 19 20
11-12 PM	3 4 5 6 7 8 9 10 11 12 13 14 15 16 17 18 19 20	3 4 5 6 7 8 9 10 11 12 13 14 15 16 17 18 19 20	3 4 5 6 7 8 9 10 11 12 13 14 15 16 17 18 19 20	3 4 5 6 7 8 9 10 11 12 13 14 15 16 17 18 19 20	3 4 5 6 7 8 9 10 11 12 13 14 15 16 17 18 19 20	3 4 5 6 7 8 9 10 11 12 13 14 15 16 17 18 19 20	3 4 5 6 7 8 9 10 11 12 13 14 15 16 17 18 19 20
12-1 PM	3 4 5 6 7 8 9 10 11 12 13 14 15 16 17 18 19 20	3 4 5 6 7 8 9 10 11 12 13 14 15 16 17 18 19 20	3 4 5 6 7 8 9 10 11 12 13 14 15 16 17 18 19 20	3 4 5 6 7 8 9 10 11 12 13 14 15 16 17 18 19 20	3 4 5 6 7 8 9 10 11 12 13 14 15 16 17 18 19 20	3 4 5 6 7 8 9 10 11 12 13 14 15 16 17 18 19 20	3 4 5 6 7 8 9 10 11 12 13 14 15 16 17 18 19 20
1-2 PM	3 4 5 6 7 8 9 10 11 12 13 14 15 16 17 18 19 20	3 4 5 6 7 8 9 10 11 12 13 14 15 16 17 18 19 20	3 4 5 6 7 8 9 10 11 12 13 14 15 16 17 18 19 20	3 4 5 6 7 8 9 10 11 12 13 14 15 16 17 18 19 20	3 4 5 6 7 8 9 10 11 12 13 14 15 16 17 18 19 20	3 4 5 6 7 8 9 10 11 12 13 14 15 16 17 18 19 20	3 4 5 6 7 8 9 10 11 12 13 14 15 16 17 18 19 20
2-3 PM	3 4 5 6 7 8 9 10 11 12 13 14 15 16 17 18 19 20	3 4 5 6 7 8 9 10 11 12 13 14 15 16 17 18 19 20	3 4 5 6 7 8 9 10 11 12 13 14 15 16 17 18 19 20	3 4 5 6 7 8 9 10 11 12 13 14 15 16 17 18 19 20	3 4 5 6 7 8 9 10 11 12 13 14 15 16 17 18 19 20	3 4 5 6 7 8 9 10 11 12 13 14 15 16 17 18 19 20	3 4 5 6 7 8 9 10 11 12 13 14 15 16 17 18 19 20
3-4 PM	3 4 5 6 7 8 9 10 11 12 13 14 15 16 17 18 19 20	3 4 5 6 7 8 9 10 11 12 13 14 15 16 17 18 19 20	3 4 5 6 7 8 9 10 11 12 13 14 15 16 17 18 19 20	3 4 5 6 7 8 9 10 11 12 13 14 15 16 17 18 19 20	3 4 5 6 7 8 9 10 11 12 13 14 15 16 17 18 19 20	3 4 5 6 7 8 9 10 11 12 13 14 15 16 17 18 19 20	3 4 5 6 7 8 9 10 11 12 13 14 15 16 17 18 19 20
4-5 PM	3 4 5 6 7 8 9 10 11 12 13 14 15 16 17	3 4 5 6 7 8 9 10 11 12 13 14 15 16 17	3 4 5 6 7 8 9 10 11 12 13 14 15 16 17	3 4 5 6 7 8 9 10 11 12 13 14 15 16 17	3 4 5 6 7 8 9 10 11 12 13 14 15 16 17	3 4 5 6 7 8 9 10 11 12 13 14 15 16 17	3 4 5 6 7 8 9 10 11 12 13 14 15 16 17

	18 19 20	18 19 20	18 19 20	18 19 20	18 19 20	18 19 20	18 19 20
5-6 PM	3 4 5 6 7 8 9 10 11 12 13 14 15 16 17 18 19 20	3 4 5 6 7 8 9 10 11 12 13 14 15 16 17 18 19 20	3 4 5 6 7 8 9 10 11 12 13 14 15 16 17 18 19 20	3 4 5 6 7 8 9 10 11 12 13 14 15 16 17 18 19 20	3 4 5 6 7 8 9 10 11 12 13 14 15 16 17 18 19 20	3 4 5 6 7 8 9 10 11 12 13 14 15 16 17 18 19 20	3 4 5 6 7 8 9 10 11 12 13 14 15 16 17 18 19 20
6-7 PM	3 4 5 6 7 8 9 10 11 12 13 14 15 16 17 18 19 20	3 4 5 6 7 8 9 10 11 12 13 14 15 16 17 18 19 20	3 4 5 6 7 8 9 10 11 12 13 14 15 16 17 18 19 20	3 4 5 6 7 8 9 10 11 12 13 14 15 16 17 18 19 20	3 4 5 6 7 8 9 10 11 12 13 14 15 16 17 18 19 20	3 4 5 6 7 8 9 10 11 12 13 14 15 16 17 18 19 20	3 4 5 6 7 8 9 10 11 12 13 14 15 16 17 18 19 20
7-8 PM	3 4 5 6 7 8 9 10 11 12 13 14 15 16 17 18 19 20	3 4 5 6 7 8 9 10 11 12 13 14 15 16 17 18 19 20	3 4 5 6 7 8 9 10 11 12 13 14 15 16 17 18 19 20	3 4 5 6 7 8 9 10 11 12 13 14 15 16 17 18 19 20	3 4 5 6 7 8 9 10 11 12 13 14 15 16 17 18 19 20	3 4 5 6 7 8 9 10 11 12 13 14 15 16 17 18 19 20	3 4 5 6 7 8 9 10 11 12 13 14 15 16 17 18 19 20
8-9 PM	3 4 5 6 7 8 9 10 11 12 13 14 15 16 17 18 19 20	3 4 5 6 7 8 9 10 11 12 13 14 15 16 17 18 19 20	3 4 5 6 7 8 9 10 11 12 13 14 15 16 17 18 19 20	3 4 5 6 7 8 9 10 11 12 13 14 15 16 17 18 19 20	3 4 5 6 7 8 9 10 11 12 13 14 15 16 17 18 19 20	3 4 5 6 7 8 9 10 11 12 13 14 15 16 17 18 19 20	3 4 5 6 7 8 9 10 11 12 13 14 15 16 17 18 19 20
9-10 PM	3 4 5 6 7 8 9 10 11 12 13 14 15 16 17 18 19 20	3 4 5 6 7 8 9 10 11 12 13 14 15 16 17 18 19 20	3 4 5 6 7 8 9 10 11 12 13 14 15 16 17 18 19 20	3 4 5 6 7 8 9 10 11 12 13 14 15 16 17 18 19 20	3 4 5 6 7 8 9 10 11 12 13 14 15 16 17 18 19 20	3 4 5 6 7 8 9 10 11 12 13 14 15 16 17 18 19 20	3 4 5 6 7 8 9 10 11 12 13 14 15 16 17 18 19 20
10-11 PM	3 4 5 6 7 8 9 10 11 12 13 14 15 16 17 18 19 20	3 4 5 6 7 8 9 10 11 12 13 14 15 16 17 18 19 20	3 4 5 6 7 8 9 10 11 12 13 14 15 16 17 18 19 20	3 4 5 6 7 8 9 10 11 12 13 14 15 16 17 18 19 20	3 4 5 6 7 8 9 10 11 12 13 14 15 16 17 18 19 20	3 4 5 6 7 8 9 10 11 12 13 14 15 16 17 18 19 20	3 4 5 6 7 8 9 10 11 12 13 14 15 16 17 18 19 20
11-12 AM	3 4 5 6 7 8 9 10 11 12 13 14 15 16 17 18 19 20	3 4 5 6 7 8 9 10 11 12 13 14 15 16 17 18 19 20	3 4 5 6 7 8 9 10 11 12 13 14 15 16 17 18 19 20	3 4 5 6 7 8 9 10 11 12 13 14 15 16 17 18 19 20	3 4 5 6 7 8 9 10 11 12 13 14 15 16 17 18 19 20	3 4 5 6 7 8 9 10 11 12 13 14 15 16 17 18 19 20	3 4 5 6 7 8 9 10 11 12 13 14 15 16 17 18 19 20

At the top of the chart, circle the day(s) that you are committed to work on improving your flexibility. Then in the column 1, circle the time(s) of day that you are committed to work on improving your flexibility. Finally, in the box corresponding to the day(s) and time(s) that you are committed to, circle the number of minutes that you are committed to working on flexibility.

Figure 8.9—Determining Your Level of Commitment

DETERMINING YOUR LEVEL OF COMMITMENT TO BEING MORE FLEXIBLE

How committed are you to working on your flexibility? How many days per week and minutes per workout will you commit to improving your flexibility?   1 2 3 4 5 6 7 8 9

So where are you on the commitment scale?

1	**2**	**3**	**4**	**5**	**6**	**7**	**8**	**9**
Low commitment				**Moderate Commitment**			**High Commitment**	

The most important factor in developing and eventually maintaining a high level of commitment is to find the time that fits for you. Instead of changing around your lifestyle to find the time to work on flexibility, simply write down the available time you have right now. You are better off having a high level of commitment to work on flexibility two times per week than a low level of commitment to work on flexibility five times per week. As the weeks' progress and you are experiencing the many benefits associated with being more flexible, you will inevitably find some more time to continue improving you flexibility. See Figure 8.9 to determine the day(s), time(s) and number of minutes you are committed to working on flexibility.

Spicing Up Your Flexibility Program

In order to make your flexibility program fun, enjoyable and something you look forward to doing, there are a few strategies for you to consider while stretching.

1. First, determine the environment/location where you would like to stretch.

   A. *At home (inside)*—This may be the perfect place for you if you find comfort in just thinking about going home after school or work. Simply pick a comfortable place where you can stand, sit, and lie down and you are ready.

   B. *At home outside (backyard)*—Perhaps you prefer to be outside, and you have a great outdoor spot to stretch of your house. If so, take a mat, towel or blanket out with you and do your flexibility exercises in that favorite spot (weather permitting of course).

   C. *Local gym*—If you belong to a gym and exercise there, then consider adding a few minutes to your workout for stretching. Here are a few strategies for you to consider: (1) stretch after your CRE workout; (2) stretch in between sets and after your muscular fitness workout; (3) stretch after you warm up; (4) take your exercise prescription for flexibility with you and stretch as a total body workout rather than as a warm up or cool down; (5) sign up for a Yoga class and get your stretching done there;

D. *At work*—Perhaps you work a long hard day and by the time you come home you are tired, achy, and lack the motivation to do any physical activity. If that is your situation, then consider finding some time to stretch at work. You could come to work a few minutes early, stay a few minutes late or find some time in between (e.g., lunch hour, schedule a 10 minute appointment for yourself).

E. *Scenic place*—If you are someone who loves nature and is motivated to be in a beautiful, naturalistic setting, then consider a nice park, beach or aesthetically appealing location to do your stretches.

2. With whom do you like to stretch?

A. *By yourself*—If you like to workout alone, then schedule a time and place where you can be by yourself (e.g., home, office, large outdoor facility, gym during down time) to stretch. If you are very busy and have a full day of classes or appointments with few or no breaks in between, then you should consider scheduling an appointment with yourself a day or two in advance to stretch for a few minutes.

B. *With a partner*—If you are motivated to work on your flexibility with a partner then you should consider enrolling in a college or university exercise class. Believe it or not, many students enroll in exercise classes to find someone with similar interests. If you are not a university student, you might be able to take a fitness class in a continuing education program. If you are not connected to a university, you might consider joining a local gym. Inquire from some of the other members if they are looking for someone to stretch with. Finally, if you do not belong to either, how about enrolling a friend, neighbor, co-worker or significant other to stretch with you?

   Once you find a partner with whom to stretch, make sure your schedules are compatible. Each of you should write time the days and times that you have free to stretch together. Once you have a fit, then identify the location where you will stretch together. Make the commitment to each other that once you write down your "flexibility schedule" you are no longer "flexible" to change it. Of course, emergencies do happen and therefore you should always have a back-up plan that if for any reason you cannot stick to your assigned schedule, you will immediately contact your partner and reschedule.

3. What ambiance/atmosphere motivates you most to want to stretch?

A. *Music*—If you like music, then create your own stretching CD and put your favorite songs together to listen to while stretching. Your mind will be free to wander and take away any negative thoughts you might have about stretching. If, on the other hand, you prefer quiet, then find a time and place where you can be alone and free from noise or interaction from others-perhaps, at work before anyone else arrives or after everyone has left, or, at home once everyone has left for the day or gone to sleep.

    B. *Television*—If you are a television buff and have several favorite shows that you watch regularly, then maybe you should stretch during a segment of these shows or during the commercials.

    C. *Conversation*—If you are a frequent talker and on the phone a lot, then maybe you should plan to stretch while you have a conversation with someone

   4. Finally, if you are goal-oriented then set some SMAART flexibility goals (see below).

SETTING SMAART GOALS TO IMPROVE YOUR FLEXIBILITY

In order to increase your motivation and commitment to be more flexible, you should set SMAART goals. You can use any of the four components of your exercise prescription to set your SMAART goals. Simply ask yourself, "What motivates me the most to want to work on flexibility frequency? intensity? time? or type? Let's use Stan as an example of how to set SMAART goals using F-I-T-T.

F	Stan's goal is to stretch three times this week on Monday, Wednesday, & Friday at the campus exercise facility.
I	Stan's goal is to reach his toes on the sitting toe touch stretch.
T	Stan's goal is to stretch for 20 minutes this week and hold each stretch for at least 16 seconds.
T	Stan's first goal is to find a partner and do two PNF stretches this week. Stan's second goal is to do five static stretches per workout. He will stretch the following muscle groups: quadriceps, hamstrings, hip flexors, triceps, neck, back.

As you can see, Stan has incorporated the SMAART principle in the following manner: He has identified *specific* muscle groups that he wants to work (e.g., quadriceps, hamstrings, hip flexors, etc). His goals are clearly *measurable* in several ways: (1) stretch three times per week; (2) reach his toes on the toe touch stretch; (3) stretch for 20 minutes per week; (4) hold each stretch for 16 seconds; (5) find a partner to stretch with and (6) perform five static stretches per workout; He has an *action plan* of where the stretching will take place and what types of stretching will be done. His goals can easily be *adjusted* in the event that they will not be reached (e.g., three times to two times per week; stretch at home). His goals seem *realistic,* however, it may take Stan a week or two to determine just how close he is towards reaching his/her weekly goals and how realistic the goal really actually is. Finally, Stan has a *time frame* of stretching 20 minutes in a week. So remember that in order for you be motivated and stay committed to improve your flexibility, you need to, "STRETCH SMAART."

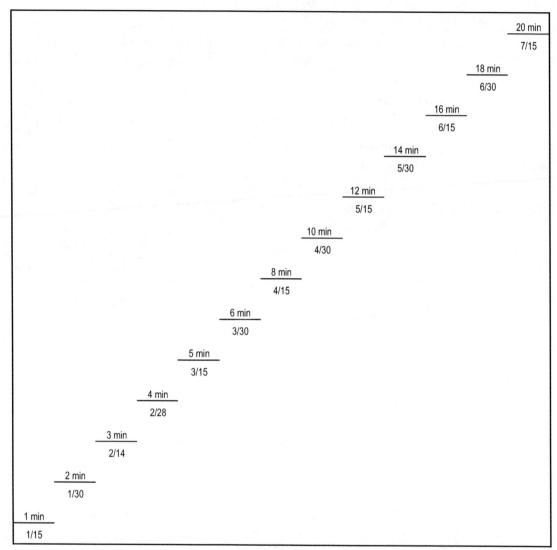

To use the Stairway to Success effectively, start out by using the bottom step to record your present performance (e.g., 1 min). Then use the top step to record your dream goal (20 min). Then go back to the second step from the bottom. That is your first short term goal (stretch for 2 minutes by 1/30). When you reach that goal, then you set a goal on the next step and so on. If at any time you do not reach your short term goal, determine what stopped you and then incorporate the strategies you have learned to get back in action and climb the stairs toward your next goal.

Figure 8.10—Using Staircase Goals to Increase Total Minutes Stretching

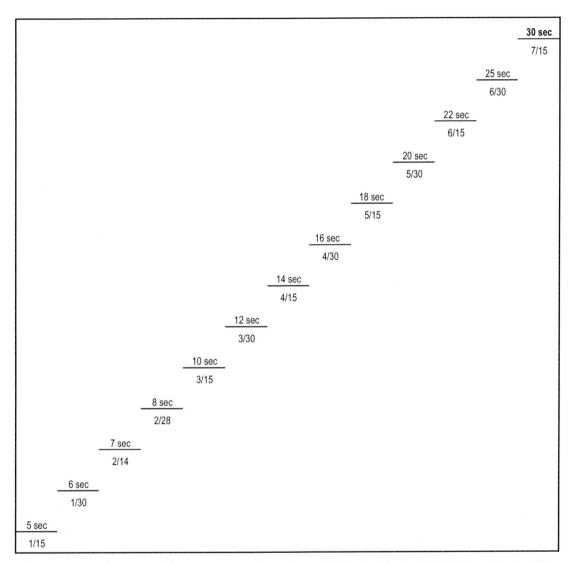

The bottom step is used to record the present number of seconds a stretch is being held for at the beginning of the flexibility program. (e.g., 5 seconds on 1/15). The top represents the long term goal of holding a stretch for 30 seconds to be achieved by 7/15. The second step from the bottom is your first short term goal (stretch for 2 minutes by 1/30). When you reach that goal, then you set a goal on the next step and so on. If at any time you do not reach your short-term goal, determine what stopped you and then incorporate the strategies you have learned to get back in action and climb the stairs toward your next goal.

Figure 8.11—Using Staircase Goals to Increase Length of Time Holding a Stretch

Another way to increase your motivation using Goal Setting is to use the Staircase. Figure 8.10 demonstrates how Debbie used the Staircase to set goals for minutes in a single workout or a full week, and Figure 8.11 shows how Jeff used the Staircase to set goals for how long he wanted to hold a stretch.

In the example used in Figure 8.10, Debbie started out stretching for 1 minute on January 15. Her long term goal was to be able to stretch for 20 minutes by July 15. Every two weeks, Debbie set a short term goal to improve her performance by stretching one to two minutes longer than she did in the previous week. Each time she reached her short-term goal, Debbie moved one step up the staircase, getting closer and closer to her long-term goal of stretching for 20 minutes. And before she knew it, Debbie's long-term dream goal of climbing up all of the stairs became nothing more than a single, short-term goal. Use Appendix 8B to create your own Stairway to Success goals if you want to increase the length of time you would like to stretch each week.

In Figure 8.11 Jeff used the staircase to set a goal for how long he wanted to be able to hold a stretch for. As of January 15, Jeff could only hold a stretch for five seconds while his long-term goal was to be able to hold a stretch for 30 seconds by 7/15. Jeff's first goal was to be able to hold a stretch for 6 seconds and he wanted to achieve that by 1/30. Each time Jeff achieved his short-term goal, he set a more challenging goal up the staircase, until he too reach his long-term goal of holding each of his stretches for 30 seconds each. Use Appendix 8C to create your own Stairway to Success goals if you want to improve holding each stretch longer.

INCORPORATING THE PRINCIPLES
OF CONDITIONING INTO YOUR FLEXIBILITY PROGRAM

Warm Up Principle—Working on your flexibility means more than just stretching as a warm-up for other activities. To prepare your muscles to be stretched properly and efficiently, you have to warm them up first. Otherwise you will increase your chance of injury and feel discomfort while stretching. An effective way to warm up before stretching is to activate "your working muscles"—the muscles you are planning to stretch. For lower leg muscles (hamstring, quadricep, calf, hip flexor), you can start out by selecting any large muscle activity (e.g., walking, jogging, riding a bike) and do it at a light intensity for a few minutes. For your upper body (arms, chest, back, shoulders), you can model some of the resistance training exercises without weights (e.g., tricep extension, bench press, lat pull down, front raises) and move your body in the exact same way you would if you were lifting weights. This will warm up these areas and facilitate your stretches.

Principle of Progression—To satisfy this principle for flexibility, you must specify how you will improve your flexibility during your workouts. You can use any of the four components from your exercise prescription to systematically show your progress. For example, you can increase your Frequency by going from two to three days per week. You can increase your Intensity by achieving a more challenging tension point (e.g., stretching from your ankles to your toes on a sit and reach stretch). You can improve Time by stretching for a longer period. For example, if you were able to hold your stretches for eight seconds in Week 1, you can strive to hold for 10 seconds in Week 2. If you stretched for a total of five minutes in Week 1, you can add increase to six minutes in Week 2. Finally, you can improve Type by adding more stretches or incorporating different flexibility techniques into your program. For example, say you began with four different static stretches in Week 1. In week 2, you might add one PNF and one passive static stretch to your workout for a total of six stretches.

Principle of Individuality—Whether you decide to stretch by yourself, with a partner or in a small group, you must focus on your own level of flexibility and not compare your performance with that of anybody else. Be proud of getting started and recognize that your progress is bound to happen provided you do one simple thing: Stick to your program.

Principle of Fun—Several ways to incorporate the principle of fun into your flexibility program are: (1) find a comfortable place to stretch; (2) stretch to music that makes you feel good; (3) stretch while watching your favorite TV shows; (4) stretch with a partner or significant other; (4) stretch with your goals in mind.

Principle of Reversibility—To avoid going backwards, you have to stick to your program. Focus on when you will stretch each week, where, with whom, and for how long. If for any reason, you do not stick to your program, immediately identify what stopped you and incorporate a strategy to increase your motivation (set SMAART goals, change your environment, listen to music, etc). Ideally, it is best if you can incorporate a few flexibility workouts per week into your schedule. However, if that is not practical for you, then consider incorporating stretching exercises into your CRE and muscular fitness exercise routines. For example, before your begin your CRE workout, warm up for a few minutes by performing your aerobic activity at a light intensity. Then stretch for a few minutes. Not only will this make your muscles feel better, it will also improve the quality of your workout. Then when you complete your CRE activity, stretch again to decrease muscle soreness and tension caused by your exercise overload. When working on muscular fitness, you can stretch in between sets to reduce any tension commonly caused by overloading your muscles. Another suggestion to consider is that you can take a few minutes out of your daily schedule and work on a few exercises either at home before bed, when you wake up, in between commercials or while you are on the telephone or computer.

Principle of Specificity—In order to make sure you are using the principle of specificity properly, be sure you know which stretches you intend to do and what your tension point is. Always stretch to the point of tension and hold; remember that pain and tension are not synonymous. Tension is a good sign. It means that you are overloading your muscles and increasing your range of motion which will ultimately make you feel better. Pain is bad and could be a sign that you are overdoing it a bit and risking possible injury. Finally, if you are stretching as a warm up or cool down from another activity, you should be stretching the muscles that you plan to or already have worked on.

EVALUATING THE SUCCESS OF YOUR FLEXIBILITY PROGRAM

Have you followed your exercise prescription? Are you as committed as you thought you would be? Do you see any improvements from Week 1 to Week 4? Use Table 8.2 to evaluate the success of your flexibility program.

Table 8.2
Evaluating the Success of Your Flexibility Program

1. Have you achieved success in the following areas?
   a. number of days you work on flexibility   YES   NO
   b. number of minutes stretched in a daily workout   YES   NO
   c. number of minutes stretched in a week   YES   NO
   d. number of exercises being incorporated into your flexibility workout
      YES   NO
   e. reaching new tension points   YES   NO

2. Has you level of motivation to work on flexibility increased, decreased or remained the same during the past four weeks
      INCREASED   DECREASED   REMANED THE SAME

3. Compare how you felt on the days you worked on flexibility with the days you did not.
      FELT BETTER   FELT WORSE   FELT THE SAME

4. How did you feel about setting and focusing on you staircase goals?

5. Describe the effect that your goals had on your flexibility performance and enjoyment.

6. Has you level of commitment to continue working on improving your flexibility
      INCREASED   DECREASED   REMANED THE SAME

If you answered "NO" to any of these questions then you should determine what is stopping you and develop a plan of action to overcome these barriers and get back on track. See Figure 8.12 to discover what, if anything is stopping you.

What is Stopping You?

Boredom	Doesn't fit into my schedule
No Results	Cannot find a partner
No Fun	Too painful
Inconvenient	Not sure what to do
Other	

Circle all of the possible barriers you have discovered for not following your flexibility exercise prescription (FEP). Then take a few moments and create a strategy to overcome each of your identified barriers and ***get back into action.*** Remember, even if you commit to only one day per week, as long as it fits into your schedule then it's the right start for you.

Strategy 1 _____

_____

_____

Strategy 2 _____

_____

_____

Strategy 3 _____

_____

_____

Strategy 4 _____

_____

_____

Strategy 5 _____

_____

_____

Figure 8.12—What is Stopping You?

As long as you are highly committed to improving your flexibility, then you will continue to search for the all the ways your flexibility exercise prescription will fit into your life. Remember, commitment does not mean that you will always reach your goals. It does mean, however, that you will never stop in your quest to improve and be proud of your efforts to live a healthy lifestyle. Please fill out Table 8.3 to discover the benefits you have achieved by working on your flexibility.

Table 8.3
Determining the Benefits of Working on Your Flexibility

1. After I stretch I feel   better   worse

2. Stretching is   relaxing   stressful

3. Stretching helps/does not help my productivity in other forms of exercise (e.g., CRE, MF)

4. Has stretching had any affect on injury frequency or severity

5. As a result of working on my flexibility over the past 1-2-3-4 weeks, I am more motivated to spend time stretching   yes   no

6. I enjoy stretching

       1   2   3   4   5   6   7   8   9
   Not at all   Very much

7. If I get stopped from sticking with my flexibility program, I will incorporate the following strategies to increase my commitment: (Circle all possibilities)

     enroll a partner to stretch with me

     set goals for frequency, intensity, time or type to keep me focused on stretching

     listen to music

     set aside time to stretch

     write down when I will stretch

     consider several places that motivate me to want to stretch (backyard, local park, gym, office, etc).

     other

PREVENTING INJURIES

One of the most effective ways to reduce and prevent injuries is to work on your flexibility. There are several guidelines that you should incorporate in order to get the best stretch and they are:

1. Warm up before stretching
2. Use flexibility as a workout rather than only a warm up or cool down
3. Stretch after you cool down
4. Learn correct form while stretching

5. Learn where your tension points are

6. Stretch to a point of tension, not pain

7. Stretch slowly and gently

8. Avoid overstretching

9. Avoid bouncing

This chapter introduced you to muscular flexibility and explained the importance of incorporating flexibility exercises into your lifestyle. A variety of flexibility assessments (e.g., formal and informal) and exercises have been introduced so that you can determine how flexible you are and assist you in designing a flexibility exercise prescription that is just right for you. In addition, several strategies are introduced to spice up your flexibility workouts and create a fun and productive atmosphere that will help you to look forward to working on your flexibility. Finally, guidelines to prevent injuries are listed to help you exercise safely. So be a little flexible and find the time to stretch it out!

REVIEW QUESTIONS

1. Define flexibility.

2. List five benefits of being flexible and explain which one(s) mean the most to you?

3. Describe two ways to assess your flexibility

4. List four different flexibility techniques and explain the benefits and limitations of each?

5. Which technique(s) do you like the most? least? and why?

6. What are some common problems people have when stretching? What solutions can you offer to prevent these problems from occurring?

7. Explain why you should avoid working on flexibility only as a warm up to other activities?

8. How can you measure F-I-T-T for your flexibility program?

9. List three to five ways to spice up your flexibility program. Which one(s) work for you?

10. Create one to two S-M-A-A-R-T that can help you to improve your flexibility?

11. Explain how you have incorporated the principles of conditioning into your flexibility program?

12. How successful is your flexibility program?

13. What can you do to make your flexibility exercise program even more successful?

14. List four ways to prevent injuries while stretching.

LAB ASSIGNMENT 8.1

Questions 1-10 should be answered prior to beginning your Flexibility Exercise Program.

1. How committed are you to improving your flexibility over the next four weeks?

    low   moderate   high

2. If you have a low level of commitment, what strategies will you incorporate to increase your level of commitment to improve your flexibility?

3. List your SMAART goals for improving your flexibility over the next four weeks?

    A. _____

    B. _____

    C. _____

4. Using the stairway to success, convert your SMAART goals into stairway goals over the next four weeks.

5. Develop an exercise prescription to improve your flexibility over the next 4 weeks.

	Week 1	Week 2	Week 3	Week 4
F				
I				
T				
T				

* For intensity—list each exercise and your present tension point in Week 1 and your desired tension points (where you are striving to get to in Weeks' 2-4. For Type, list the exercises you plan to use to improve your flexibility as well as the flexibility techniques (e.g., static, passive static, PNF) you are considering.

6. Explain how you will be satisfying the principle of progression over the next four weeks.

7. Describe how you plan to incorporate the principle of recuperation into your flexibility program?

8. How do you plan to satisfy the warm up principle prior to working on your flexibility?

9. What strategies are you considering to incorporate the principle of fun into your flexibility workouts?

10. What strategies do you have planned to avoid the principle of reversibility?

Questions 11-14 should be answered at the conclusion of each week.

11. Explain how you have been overloading from Weeks' 1 to Week 4?

12. How successful were you in avoiding the principle of reversibility?

13. How much have your improved from Weeks' 1 to Week 4?

14. Did you have fun while working on your flexibility? If so, explain the strategies that you have incorporated to have fun. If you did not have fun, explain what you plan to do over the next few weeks to make your flexibility workouts more fun (e.g., music, exercising with a partner, etc).

REFERENCES AND RECOMMENDED READINGS

American College of Sports Medicine (1998). Position Stand: The recommended quantity and quality of exercise for developing and maintaining cardiorespiratory and muscular fitness and flexibility in healthy adults. *Medicine and Science in Sports and Exercise, 30*, 975-991.

Alter, M.J. (1996). Science of Stretching, Human Kinetics: Champaign, IL.

Bowles, H.R., Morrow, J.R., Jr., Leonard, B.L., Hawkins, M., & Couzelis, P.M. (2002). The association between physical activity behavior and commonly reported barriers in a worksite population. *Research Quarterly for Exercise and Sport, 73,* 464-470.

Bracko, M.R. (2002). Can stretching prior to exercise and sports improve performance and prevent injury? *ACSM's Health and Fitness Journal, 6*(5), 17-22.

Corbin, C., Welk, G., Corbin, W., & Welk, K. (2006). Concepts of physical fitness: Active lifestyles for wellness, pp 160 13th edition. McGraw Hill

Hoeger, W.K. & Hoeger, S.A. (2004). Principles & labs for fitness and wellness 7th edition. pp 226-246. Thomson:Wadsworth.

Knudsen, D.V. (2002). Stretchig during warm-up: Do we have enough evidence? *Journal of Physical Education, Recreation, and Dance, 70,* 271-277.

Liemohn, W.P. (2003). Exercise prescription for flexibility and low-back function. *In Health Fitness Instructor's Handbook.* 4th ed. E.T. Howley and B.D. Franks (eds). Human Kinetics: Champaign, IL.

McAtee, R.E. & Charland, J. (1993). Facilitated stretching, 2nd edition. Human Kinetics: Champaign, IL.

Morrow, Jr, J.R., Krzewinski-Malone, J.A., Jackson, A.W., Bungun, T., & FitzGerald. S.J. (2004). American adults' knowledge of exercise recommendations. *Research Quarterly for Exercise and Sport, 75,* 3, 231-237.

APPENDIX 8A
FLEXIBILITY WORKOUT CARD

Flexibility Exercise		Day 1	Day 2	Day 3	Day 4	Day 5	Day 6	Day 7
	Sec Held Sets TP							
	Sec Held Sets TP							
	Sec Held Sets TP							
	Sec Held Sets TP							
	Sec Held Sets TP							
	Sec Held Sets TP							
	Sec Held Sets TP							
	Sec Held Sets TP							
	Sec Held Sets TP							
Goal	Sec Held Sets TP							

Record the number of seconds you hold each stretch in the sec held column;
TP stands for tension point. Each time you stretch record your tension point.
In the Goal Row, you can set goals for hold long you want to hold a stretch for and what tension point you would like to achieve. Use Day 1 as your baseline and set goals starting in day 2.

APPENDIX 8B
STAIRCASE GOALS FOR STRETCHING LONGER DAILY OR WEEKLY

Start out by using the bottom step to record the present total of minutes you stretch for each day or week (e.g., 1 min). Then use the top step to record your dream goal of how many minutes you would like to stretch for 6 months from the date that you started stretching. Then go back to the second step from the bottom and set your first short term goal of how many minutes you would like to be able to stretch for approximately two weeks from your starting date. When you reach that goal, you can set your next short-term goal on the next step above and so on. If at any time you do not reach your short term goal, determine what stopped you and then incorporate the strategies you have learned to get back in action and climb the stairs toward your next goal.

APPENDIX 8C
STAIRCASE GOALS FOR HOLDING YOUR STRETCHES LONGER

Start out by using the bottom step to record the number of seconds you currently hold a stretch for. Then use the top step to record your long-term dream goal of how long you would like to be able to hold a stretch for 6 months for the date that you started stretching. Then go back to the second step from the bottom and set your first short term goal of how many seconds you would like to be able to hold a stretch for approximately two weeks from your starting date. When you reach that goal, you can set your next short-term goal on the next step above and so on. If at any time you do not reach your short-term goal, determine what stopped you and then incorporate the strategies you have learned to get back in action and climb the stairs toward your next goal.

Chapter 9

Eating Healthy

OBJECTIVES

After this chapter, you will be able to:

- identify what poor eating is and what motivates you to eat this way
- learn what healthy eating really is
- distinguish between the Old Food Guide Pyramid and the New Food Guide Pyramid
- learn the functions of the six basic nutrients
- implement strategies to eat healthier foods
- determine your level of commitment to healthy eating
- set S-M-A-A-R-T goals to improve your nutritional habits
- evaluate the success of your present eating habits

- "I don't have time."
- "I'm just not hungry for breakfast."
- "I have to have my coffee in the morning."
- "It just doesn't taste as good without the extra cheese."
- "I never eat lunch."
- "I eat whenever I'm hungry."
- "But I'm hungry late at night."
- "I can't stop eating when I'm hungry."
- "It looks too good to pass up."
- "Just one more and then I'll stop."

Years ago, many people believed that eating a good meal meant eating a lot of food and the more you ate, the better the meal. Back then, many adults simply did not know what a healthy meal consisted of and terms like "balanced diet," "fat free food," "complex carbs," "plant-based," "polyunsaturated" were rarely heard. Today, one hears these words and other related words every day. The fact is most people today know how to eat healthy, yet they choose not to.

As a result of the industrial and technological revolutions, the problem has shifted from having a lack of food to consuming too much of it. Today, most people can go to the supermarket or local grocery and in less than an hour take home enough food to last at least a week. Moreover, because of the pace of life in modern society, fast food appears to have shifted from a novelty to a necessity. According to the U.S. Department of Health and Human Services, two-thirds of adults in the United States (ages 20 and older) are overweight and over 30 percent are considered obese. Alarmingly, this number is not limited to adults. The percent of young people (ages 6-19) who are overweight has tripled since 1980 (over 9 million) to over 16 percent resulting in an increased risk for many lifestyle illnesses (e.g., heart disease, cancer, obesity, atherosclerosis, high blood pressure, diabetes) (1-http://www.cdc.gov/nccdphp/dnpa/obesity.).

Today, we have a wealth of information at our disposal about how to eat healthy and maintain proper body weight. Courses in nutrition, fitness, and wellness are offered on the collegiate level, and proper eating habits are taught in health classes as early as elementary school. Unfortunately, this has not seemed to decrease poor eating habits.

Two important questions for you are:

1. Do you know how to eat healthy?

2. Do you eat healthy?

If you are like most people, then your answers are that you probably know how to eat healthy, but you do not—at least not all the time. The next question is why? Why is it that you know how to eat healthy and yet you choose not to?

WHY DO YOU EAT POORLY?

Most people know that fruits and vegetables are better than candy and ice cream. They know that baked, grilled and boiled are better than fried. They know that drinking water is better than drinking soda or alcohol. They know that eating breakfast is better than snacking a few minutes before bedtime. Yet, if you ask someone you know if he/she eats healthy, for every one person that says "yes," you will most probably find at least one person and probably more that says "no."

The fact is that people eat poorly because they are more motivated to eat that way than they are to eat healthy. They would rather give in to their cravings for the foods and drinks that they love (e.g., fast foods, candy, cake, soda), regardless of how unhealthy they are because they have become attached to eating this way. Consequently, this often results in people rationalizing or explaining their motives to eat poorly in order to reduce the guilt that is commonly associated with poor eating. Does this ring a bell for you? Here are a few common reasons that people give for eating poorly.

1. ***Poor Planning/Not enough time***—One of the most popular reasons for eating poorly is the "perception" that eating healthy foods takes more time. Many people eat "on the run," and substitute healthy food for fast food.

2. ***Develop bad eating habits from an early age***—If you grew up eating poorly then you may have acquired some bad habits (e.g., overeating, eating too many foods high in fat content, snacking on candy, eating late at night, skipping meals). Moreover, you may have become attached to these foods and find it hard to be without them (e.g., soda coffee, cheese, butter, french fries, ice cream, fast foods, candy).

3. ***Attraction to Food Ads***—How often have you seen a famous person or an attractive model endorsing a food product? You go to the store and when you see that product, an immediate image of the star that you like pops into your head and persuades you to buy it and give it a try.

4. ***Emotional attachment***—Some people eat more when they are stressed or upset. For these people, food helps to temporarily overcome negative mood states. However, these negative emotions often become exacerbated with other negative feelings such as guilt, anger, and frustration for succumbing to poor eating habits.

5. ***Psychological hunger***—Sometimes you may think you are hungry when you really are not; you prompt yourself to satisfy a psychological instinct (e.g., just one more piece) and ignore physical cues (e.g., I am full). For example, you may be full from a meal, yet continue to eat because there is still more food on your plate. You may think you are hungry in places that you frequently store food (e.g., car, living room, bedroom, classroom, briefcase, book bag), regardless of whether or not you have just eaten. When you watch TV and see commercials for foods that you like, you may become tempted to eat even though are aren't hungry.

6. ***Eat too fast***—When you are in a rush and you only have a few minutes to eat, the tendency is to "eat too fast." It takes about 20 minutes for the brain to get the message from the stomach that it is getting full. Since many people eat their meals in under 20 minutes, there is a strong chance that they overeat, without realizing it because the stomach has not sent the message to the brain quite yet. Then, after about 20 minutes one may go from feeling starved to feeling bloated and recognize that too much has been eaten in one meal.

7. ***Lack of motivation***—Some people simply do not care if they eat healthy. They are more motivated to eat what they want, when they want and as much as they want then they are to be health conscious. They have developed an invincible attitude that nothing bad could ever happen to them so it is unnecessary to ever eat healthy.

8. ***Blaming others***—Sometimes, people do not take responsibility for their poor eating habits and blame others. For example, "it's mom's fault for making it." "My friends all wanted fast food and encouraged me to eat it." "Everyone around me eats this way and I just couldn't say no." What you may not realize is that it is your choice to eat

that food. Nobody makes you eat what you don't want and so blaming others for your poor eating habits is only a temporary mechanism to reduce your guilt.

EATING HEALTHY

Everywhere you look—television, newspapers, magazines, billboards—you can find advertisements about the latest fad diet or food. But in spite of all the hype, eating healthy today is no different than it was years ago. Nutritionists are still recommending that a diet that emphasizes complex carbohydrates consisting of fruits, vegetables, and whole grains is the healthiest way of eating.

The Old Food Guide Pyramid

In 1992, the U.S. Department of Agriculture (USDA) developed the Food Guide Pyramid which illustrated the recommended number of servings for five major food groups (See Figure 9.1 for the old Food Guide Pyramid). According to the USDA, adults should be getting 6-11 servings per day of bread, whole grain cereal, rice and pasta, 2-5 servings per day of vegetables, 2-4 servings of fruits, 2-3 servings per day of milk, yogurt, cheeses, meat, poultry, fish, dry beans, eggs and nuts, and fats, oils and sweets in limited amounts and servings (U.S. Department of Health and Human Services, Department of Agriculture, 2000).

What complicated the Food Guide Pyramid was the definition of a serving size. For example, 1 piece of bread, 1/2 cup of cooked rice or pasta, ¾ cup of juice, 2 to 3 ounces of cooked lean meat, and 1 ounce of cereal were all considered to be one serving. However, most people determine one serving to be the size of one full plate of food and one full glass or cup of beverage. What they do not always realize is that the amount of food on their plate and drink in their glass or cup often exceeds one real serving. In addition, if condiments like butter, sauce, sugar or oils are being used to prepare or add flavor to foods then additional calories are being added to your foods.

The main problem with the Food Guide Pyramid was that it was not being used. For whatever reason, most Americans simply did not follow the recommended guidelines. According to the Harvard School of Public Health, the information in the old food guide pyramid didn't point to healthy eating because its blueprint was based on shaky scientific evidence which barely changed over the years to reflect major advances in understanding the connection between diet and health (www.hsph.harvard.edu/nutrition source/pyramids.html). Perhaps the old food guide pyramid was not practical for people to adopt on a consistent basis. 6-11 of this, 3-5 of that, one serving size means this, another serving size means that. All this could have made it too hard to follow. Another possibility is that the Food Guide Pyramid was not being advertised enough in the right places (e.g., restaurants, supermarkets, school cafeteria). Consequently, what people may have learned in the past about eating healthy was

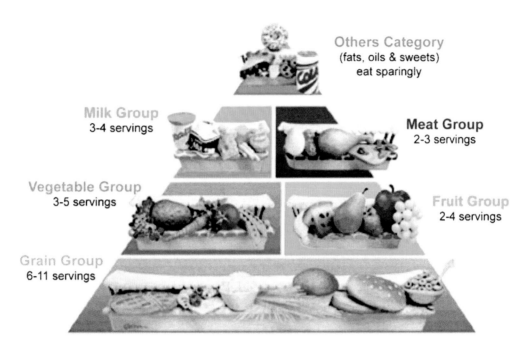

Figure 9.1—Old Food Group Pyramid

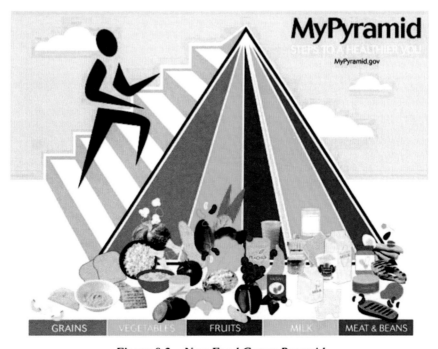

Figure 9.2—New Food Group Pyramid

quickly forgotten and replaced with the same old eating habits (e.g., consuming too many calories; consuming too much fat; skipping meals; eating late at night). For more information on the old and new food guide pyramids, you can look at www.foodguidepyramid and www.health.harvard.edu/press.

The New Food Guide Pyramid

In 2005, the U.S. government unveiled the new Food Guide Pyramid designed to address nutritional needs by shifting from one program fits all to 12 new individualized food pyramids based on one's level of physical activity (http://www.health.gov/dietary guidelines/dga 2005 document). While the old Food Guide Pyramid was horizontally based, the new pyramid is designed vertically and color coded into the following categories: (1) orange = grains; (2) green = vegetables; (3) red = fruits; (4) yellow = oils; (5) blue = milk products and (6) purple = lean meats; (See Figure 9.2 for the new Food Guide Pyramid). As you can see, the bands are different sizes with the larger bands represented by the food groups needed most to eat healthy (whole grains, vegetables and fruits). With 12 different nutritional programs, there certainly is a better chance that you might find one that fits your needs and helps you incorporate some of these guidelines into your lifestyle. It certainly beats the "one size fits all" approach of the old Food Guide Pyramid.

SIX ESSENTIAL NUTRIENTS

There are approximately 45-50 nutrients in food that are necessary for the body's growth, development, maintenance, repair and overall good health. They are classified into the following six categories: (1) carbohydrates; (2) fats; (3) proteins; (4) vitamins; (5) minerals; and (6) water. These 6 nutrients can be broken down into two more categories: ***macronutrients*** and ***micronutrients***. *Macronutrients* consist of carbohydrates, fats, and proteins, all of which are needed to provide energy for daily functions and for the building, repairing and maintenance of body tissues and organs. *Micronutrients* consist of vitamins and minerals and are needed in smaller amounts to regulate the functioning of the cells.

Carbohydrates—There are three major types of carbohydrates: (1) sugars more commonly known as simple carbohydrates; (2) starches, more common known as complex carbohydrates and (3) fiber. Simple carbohydrates have little nutritional value and are found in products like soda, cakes and candy. Complex carbohydrates are the most important nutrient and are equivalent to "premium octane gasoline." They help the body run more efficiently by providing the quickest source of energy. You can find complex carbohydrates in fruits, vegetables, whole grain breads, rice and pasta. Fiber is an indigestible carbohydrate that moves through the intestinal tract and provides bulk for feces in the large intestine, which in turn facilitates elimination. Fiber decreases the risk of cardiovascular disease and cancer and may also lower the risk of coronary heart disease. You can find fiber in fruits, legumes, oats, barley, wheat bran cereals, grains and vegetables.

Complex carbohydrates are our primary source of energy because the body is able to convert these nutrients faster than any other nutrients. When we consume carbohydrates, water is attached to it making it heavy and unable to stay that way for long. Therefore, it is just waiting to be used up. Of course, if you consume too many calories from carbohydrates, whatever is not used winds up being stored as fat. It is recommended that approximately 50-60% of your daily caloric intake come from complex carbohydrates (with no more than 10% coming from simple carbohydrates).

Isn't it interesting how many products today are advertising "low carb," "no carb" or "carb smart" as a mechanism to increase sales? Did you know that these products were made with few or no carbohydrates to begin with? They are simply being advertised to jump on the new fad that "carbs" are bad. What they do not tell you is that the body relies mostly on carbohydrates as its main source of energy especially during intense activity. In fact, the brain's major source of fuel comes in the form of glucose which comes from the breakdown of carbohydrates. Without an adequate diet of complex carbohydrates, the body is forced to use other nutrients to do their job resulting in the body overworking itself and being forced to slow down considerably due to a lack of readily available energy. For example, if you planned on running for 30-40 minutes and you consumed mostly proteins and fats with very little complex carbohydrates for the past few days, you would probably find it very difficult to complete your run. After a few minutes of running, your body would exhaust its primary source of energy (complex carbohydrates), thus making it more difficult to keep running. You may be able to push it for a little while longer, but without the complex carbohydrates in your system to fuel your workout, you would have to slow down considerably and most probably stop before the 30-40 minutes were completed.

Fats—Fats serve the following needs. First, they protect vital organs. Imagine if you had the same amount of body fat around your heart, brain or lungs that is around your kneecap. One little bang hear or there and it can cause major problems. Second, fats help to keep your body insulated and body temperature regulated. Third, fats add flavor to help you enjoy the taste of food. Finally, fats serve as the body's secondary source of energy and begin to be used as energy when you exercise for long periods of time. For example, if you consumed about 300 calories of complex carbohydrates and you are planning to exercise for a long period of time (e.g., 45 minutes or more), after 20-30 minutes, the body's readily available supply of complex carbohydrates may become depleted. Yet, what enables you to keep going is your body's ability to convert the fat that you recently ate along with some of your stored fat (the fat we all want to get rid of) to energy. An interesting way to view fats is to think of them as stored ice cubes. When you want a cold drink, you use ice with your beverage. The ice by itself will do little to quench your thirst, unless of course you want to wait an hour and let the ice melt. However, ice cools your drink more quickly, and a cold drink satisfies your thirst more efficiently. Fats in small amounts combined with carbohydrates gives the body two sources of energy that allow for longer and more efficient durations of activity.

Fats come in two forms—**saturated** and **unsaturated**. Saturated fats are found primarily in animal sources, including red meats, poultry, dairy products including egg yolks, milk and cheese as well as certain vegetable sources such as coconut and palm oils. Saturated fats are usually in a solid form and are used by the body to manufacture cholesterol. They do not melt at room temperature and therefore are not easily broken down by the body. Saturated fats are considered to be unhealthy and linked to cardiovascular disease, breast, colon, and prostate cancer and obesity. Unsaturated fats consist of two kinds: (1) **monosaturated** and (2) **polyunsaturated**. *Monosaturated* fats come primarily from vegetable sources such as olive, peanut, and canola oil. *Polyunsaturated* fats also come primarily from vegetable sources including cottonseed, soybean, safflower, sunflower and corn oils as well as cold water fish including mackerel and salmon. Both types of unsaturated fat usually come in liquid form and are considered to be healthier than saturated fat because they reduce cholesterol and can be broken down by the body and used for energy when needed. Since fats do not carry water, they can be stored in the body for long periods of time. The average American consumes over 45% of their daily caloric intake from fats (www.usda.gov; www.uhealthcare.com/topics/weight/weightcontrol). The USDA recommends that calories from fat sources should be no more than 30%. Most recently, that amount has been reduced to 15% - 25% with saturated fat only being consumed in limited amounts.

Proteins—Proteins are an important nutrient found in meats, fish, poultry, eggs, milk, cheese, and soy. Proteins serve many vital functions including: (1) enabling tissue growth; and maintaining and regulating body processes; (2) forming integral body parts including skin, tendons, ligaments, membranes, muscles, organs and bones; (3) building up of the immune system; (4) helping the body maintain fluids; (5) transporting needed substances (e.g., oxygen, minerals) and (6) providing some fuel for the body's energy needs. As an energy source, proteins rank third behind carbohydrates and fats. They are only needed for energy when the body becomes depleted of both carbohydrates and fats. For example, during times of starvation the body is forced to break down the protein in the body and use it for energy to survive because carbohydrates and fats have been depleted. Consuming large quantities of protein in place of complex carbohydrates will only force the body to use it for a job it was not meant to do. Consequently, the body will wind up overworking itself and eventually break down and function inefficiently.

Vitamins—Vitamins are organic molecules needed in small amounts to perform several bodily functions including growth, development, and metabolism. Vitamins are classified into two types: water soluble and fat soluble. Vitamins B and C are water soluble which means they dissolve in the blood and are carried to the cells. When not used, these vitamins can be excreted from the body by the kidneys. Vitamins A, D, E, and K are fat soluble which means they are stored and dissolved in fat and can stay in the body longer than water soluble vitamins. As a result, fat soluble vitamins should be taken in small quantities; otherwise they can become toxic. Since most vitamins cannot be manufactured by the body, they should be consumed on a daily basis.

Minerals—Minerals are elements needed in small amounts to help regulate a variety of bodily functions including: (1) aiding in the growth and maintenance of body tissue; (2) conduction of nerve impulses; (3) muscular contractions; (4) enzyme function (5) water balance and (6) structural functioning of bones and teeth. The major minerals that the body needs include: calcium, phosphorous, magnesium, sodium, potassium, and chloride. The trace

Table 9.1
Foods Containing Essential Vitamins and Minerals

Nutrients	
Fat Soluble Vitamins	**Where to Find**
Vitamin A	Liver, cheese, milk, yellow, orange and deep green vegetables and fruits
Vitamin D	Fortified milk, fish oils, salmon, tuna, egg yolks
Vitamin E	Vegetable oils, whole grain breads and cereals, nuts and seeds, yellow and green leafy vegetables
Vitamin K	Green leafy vegetables, eggs, cabbage, peas, potatoes, cauliflower
Water Soluble Vitamins	
Vitamin B (biotin, Folate, Niacin, Thiamin Pantothenic Acid, Roboflavin, Vitmain B6, Vitamin B12	Cereals, yeast, egg yolks, soy, flour, liver, green leafy vegetables, breads, fish, potatoes
Vitamin C	Fruits and vegetables
Minerals	**Where to Find**
Calcium	Milk and milk products, yogurt, tofu, cheese, fortified orange juice, bread, green leafy vegetables, dried beans, sardines, salmon
Copper	Seafood, meats, beans, nuts, whole grains
Iron	Meats and poultry, seafood, eggs, dried peas and beans, nuts, whole and enriched grains, green leafy vegetables, dried fruit
Phosphorous	Milk, fish, meats, eggs, whole grains, dried beans and peas, cereal.
Zinc	Milk, meat, seafood, liver, whole grains, nuts, eggs, dried beans
Magnesium	Milk, green leafy vegetables, seafood, whole grains, nuts, legumes, soybeans
Sodium	Salt, meat, processed foods
Potassium	Milk, bananas, legumes, orange juice, whole grains, potatoes, dried fruit
Selenium	Meat, seafood, eggs ,whole grains

minerals that the body needs are selenium, iron, fluoride, copper, iodine, and zinc. When you eat a balanced diet, you generally consume the majority of the minerals needed. See Table 9.1 for a list of foods containing essential vitamins and minerals.

Water—It is generally agreed that water is the single most important nutrient with approximately 50-70 percent of a person's weight being composed of water. Without water, the body cannot survive. Water is needed to: (1) transport all nutrients throughout the body; (2) carry away waste; (3) help regulate body temperature and (4) assist in the absorption and digestion of food. Each day the body loses about 2 to 3 quarts of water and in vigorous exercise and hot weather water loss is even greater. It is recommended that you drink at least 8-10 8-ounce servings of water daily.

MEASURING YOUR NUTRITIONAL INTAKE

The amount of energy present in food is measured in terms of calories. Technically, a calorie is the amount of energy needed to raise the temperature of 1 gram of water one degree Celsius. The more calories a food has, the more potential energy it has. Unfortunately, we do not get full from the number of calories or potential energy that food or drink possesses. We get full from the volume or weight of the food or beverage consumed. For example, if you ate two Pop Tarts consisting of approximately 210 calories each (420 overall) you may not be as full as if you consumed a handful of carrots, 2 apples and a banana equaling about 170 calories. Yet, if you ate a 20-ounce steak, you would get fuller than if you ate a 12 ounce steak.

There are 4 calories in 1 gram of carbohydrates, 9 calories in 1 gram of fat and 4 calories in 1 gram of protein. Therefore, you can eat 2.25 times more carbohydrates and proteins than fat for the same number of calories. In other words, fat has more potential energy to be used. However, potential energy does not mean that it is readily available or that you will even use it. As you learned in the previous section, fat is our secondary source of energy and can only be used with carbohydrates; if you do not eat enough carbohydrates, the fats will wind up sitting in your body and not be used efficiently (ice cubes without water). Nutrition experts generally agree that approximately 50-60% of your diet should consist of carbohydrates with no more than 10% coming from simple carbohydrates (sugars, candy, cake, etc), 15-25% should come from fats (predominantly monosaturated and polyunsaturated) and 15-20% from proteins.

Energy Balance Equation

A simple way to determine if you need to lose or gain weight is to use an energy balance equation which consists of two components:

1. *Energy output*—everything you do that requires energy (e.g., exercising, keeping your heart rate beating properly, keeping your body temperature regulated);

2. *Energy input*—everything that you eat and drink; When your energy output exceeds your energy input, you lose weight and when your energy input exceeds your energy output, you gain weight.

Metabolism

Your metabolism is what determines the amount of energy you will expend to keep your life sustaining systems going (respiration, circulation, digestion, temperature regulation). The faster your metabolism, the more calories you will expend at rest.

If your goal is to lose weight, the first step is to increase your energy output by becoming more physically active. (You can select the exercise programs from chapters' 6-7). Start out slow and each week commit to do just a little bit more (e.g., an extra minute or two of cardio; a few more reps on muscular fitness). Then take better control of what you eat. Become more conscious of the foods that contain little to no nutritional value. Avoid eating foods that are too high in fat (over 30% of calories coming from fat). Learn what your energy balance equation is and incorporate some of the strategies listed in the next section into your daily eating habits. You should also refer back to chapters 6-8 to see how each prescription will help you do "just a little bit more."

STRATEGIES FOR EATING HEALTHIER

If you are truly committed to eating healthy, then you should consider incorporating a few of the following strategies to help you improve. The key is to choose a strategy that fits you.

1. *Plan your meals*—Rather than waiting until you are hungry, you should plan your meal(s) a few hours to one day in advance. Decide what you are going to eat, when, where, how much, etc. For example, if you typically run out of the house early in the morning and skip breakfast, then the night before consider what you will eat for breakfast or plan to take something with you to eat in the car, bus, train or walk (e.g., fruit, sandwich) and decide at what time you will eat it. By planning your meal(s) in advance, you become less susceptible to binge eating and more resistant to eating fast food.

2. *Do not feel compelled to clean your plate* – As you begin to feel full, you should stop eating, regardless of how much food is left on your plate. Sometimes, the focus becomes finishing what is left on the plate rather than stopping when you are full. Consequently, you may overeat. By concentrating on how full you are getting, you are less likely to keep eating even though your plate still has food on it. If you want, just save the leftovers for lunch the next day.

3. *Make second helpings hard to get*—Rather than put all the food on the table when you are eating, fill your plate before you sit down and leave the remaining food in a

place where it came from (e.g., the stove, oven, counter, refrigerator). If you want a second serving, you will have to leave the table to get it. I bet that might change some of your minds from eating more.

4. ***Restrict eating to designated places***—To reduce the likelihood of overeating, restrict your eating to one or two designated places (e.g., kitchen, cafeteria) and don't put food in other places (your study or reading area, your bedroom, your living room your den or your car, for example). Eventually, you will not get hungry in places where you no longer keep food.

5. ***Shop from a list and be full***—Did you ever notice that you tend to buy more food when you shop hungry than when you are full? The more food you see, the hungrier you get and the more food you want to buy. Therefore, when you need to buy food, always remember to do three things: (1) shop from a list; (2) buy only the food on the list and (3) eat before you go shopping. This can help you to resist the temptation of buying food based on hunger rather than health.

6. ***Fork up Fork Down***—One of the most common ways of eating is what is called the "Shovel Method." You put a fork full of food in your mouth and before you have even swallowed it all you have more food on your fork ready to go into your mouth. The shovel method results in you eating too much food, too fast. Instead, consider putting your fork down on your plate until you completely chew and swallow the food that you put in your mouth. This new method will slow your rate of eating and make it easier to identify when you are getting full.

7. ***20-minutes-per-meal rule***—As you learned earlier in this chapter, it takes about 20 minutes for your brain to get the message from your stomach that you are getting full. Eating a meal in less than 20 minutes often leads to overeating so taking longer to consume an entire meal will help you recognize when you are feeling full and reduce the chances of consuming too much food at one time.

8. ***Healthy snacks***—To reduce the temptation of snacking poorly, surround yourself with healthy snacks (fruits, vegetables). Take them with you and when you begin to feel hungry, you have them right there. Eventually, this will reduce the temptation of going to the candy machine when you think you need a little snack to tide you over for a few hours.

9. ***Moderation***—If you truly love some foods that are not so healthy, it is okay to have them once in a while as long as you display some portion control. For example, is okay to have a piece of candy instead of the entire box, a few chips rather than an entire bag, a cup of ice cream instead of a big bowl. The key is moderation both in portion sizes as well as frequency. Most important, do not feel guilty about having these treats. Instead, enjoy it and recognize that it is perfectly fine to have them once in a while.

10. ***Drink Water***—Instead of drinking your calories with sodas or fruit drinks, plan to drink water. If you have trouble replacing water for soda, then try it once a day. After

you achieve this, go for twice a day, then three times, etc. Before you know it, you'll be drinking more water than soda and looking forward to it, too.

11. *Use smaller plates*—Using smaller plates makes the portion sizes seem larger and makes you think there is a lot of food on your plate. This may help you to feel fuller and reduce the amount of food you may consume in one meal.

12. *Avoid skipping meals*—When people skip meals, they often feel entitled to eat whatever they want and as much of it as they want because they are hungry. It is easy to convince yourself that it has been so long since your last meal, that the important thing is to resolve hunger pains with whatever is available, rather than to eat healthy. By taking healthy snacks with you and planning out your meals in advance, you will minimize skipping meals and reduce the chances of eating poorly.

DETERMINING YOUR LEVEL OF COMMITMENT TO BE NUTRITIOUSLY HEALTHY

How committed are you to eating and drinking healthy? Are there any strategies listed above that motivate you to improve your nutritional habits? If so, which one(s)? Remember that commitment starts from a desire to accomplish something and it is not about whether you have succeeded or failed in the past. For example, if you wanted to start eating healthy and you planned to incorporate positive nutritional habits into your daily schedule, yet for some reason you did one or more of the following:

(1) you skipped breakfast

(2) you had fast food for lunch

(3) you didn't eat any fruits or vegetables today

(4) you snacked on candy late at night.

Does that mean that you are no longer committed to eating healthy? Not necessarily! It may simply mean that you just had a bad day. Something may have stopped you from making those positive changes. Perhaps you forgot about your newly discovered commitment or maybe your bad eating habits just got the best of you. If you indeed, are truly committed to improving your eating habits, you will analyze what stopped you from sticking to your commitment to eat healthy and focus on creating other strategies that may be more realistic for you to fit into your lifestyle. Most important, stay in action. For example, plan tonight what you will eat for breakfast so this way you will not skip it in the morning. Maybe you can make your lunch tonight too or plan where you will eat to avoid eating fast food. Finally, you might want to consider taking a few healthy snacks with you (e.g., fruit) when you get hungry in between meals and erase the temptation to eat candy.

In sum, your commitment to start improving your nutritional habits is reflected in the strategies that you have considered to overcome the barriers that stopped you (e.g., eating breakfast, making your lunch, taking fruits with you for snacks) as well as the actions that you take. So take a few seconds and answer the following two questions:

How committed are you to eating and drinking healthy?
Circle the number that best represents how committed you are to eat and drink healthy. You can fill this out daily or weekly.

1   2   3   4   5   6   7   8   9

SETTING S-M-A-A-R-T GOALS TO IMPROVE YOUR NUTRITIONAL HABITS

In chapters 6-8, you learned how to use S-M-A-A-R-T goals to improve your cardio-respiratory endurance, muscular fitness, and flexibility. Now it is time to set S-M-A-A-R-T goals to improve your nutritional habits. So, instead of just thinking about why you eat poorly or that you need to improve, let's "GET SMAART." Below is an example of how to use SMAART goals to improve your nutritional habits.

S—*Specifically* determine what you want to improve (e.g., eating more fruits and vegetables; reducing caloric intake).

M—Set goal(s) that you can *measure* (e.g., total number of calories consumed on a daily basis; percent of calories coming from carbohydrates, proteins, fats; the number of meals you will plan each day; the number of glasses of water you will drink in a day).

A—Determine the *actions* will you take to reach your goals and improve your nutritional habits? For example, if you normally skip meals, you can plan one meal a day in advance (e.g., I will have a tuna sandwich for lunch at 1 PM). If you do not eat enough fruits or vegetables, you can plan ahead and determine when you will. For example, you will eat a fruit in between breakfast and lunch and then have a salad for lunch. If you overeat, you can reduce your portion sizes. If you eat too fast, you can time your meals and concentrate on eating more slowly (e.g., I will take 30 minutes to eat my lunch). Whatever your goal is, you want to have an action that will direct your efforts toward reaching it.

A—If you know that you are not going to reach your goal, then you have to make an *adjustment*. For example, if your goal was to replace soda with water one time per day and it is already Day 4 and you have not had any water this week, then you can adjust your goal by committing to drinking water one time over the next 3 days. Adjusting your goal allows you to focus on making improvements rather than giving up when you know that you cannot reach the original goal(s) set.

R—To make sure your goals are *realistic* you should set goals that are within your reach. Rather than immediately giving up all the foods that you love so much that are low in nutritional value, cut down a little at a time. Begin to replace some of the low nutrition products that you consume more out of habit and convenience with healthier choices. For instance, replacing candy and cake once per day with a piece of fruit, replacing soda with water every other day, using fat-free salad dressing instead of mayonnaise, and going from eating spontaneously to planning at least one meal per day. Setting realistic goals will help you make the transition from unhealthy to healthy in a way that works for you.

T—Establish a *time frame* to reach your goals. You can set short-term goals that focus on daily to weekly actions or long term goals that emphasize something that you want to accomplish that will take several months to achieve. For example, say you eat fast food at least five times per week and you snack on fattening products every night until you go to sleep. You drink 2-3 cans of soda per day and use butter at least twice per day on items such as muffins, bread, and vegetables. Your meals are 80 percent spontaneous and only 20 percent planned, and too often your dietary analysis indicates that you eat more than 3000 calories per day, 50 percent of which is fat calories. In the short-term, you may set a goal to replace one highly fattening product for something lower in fat as well as calories (e.g., replace muffin with butter for a bowl of oatmeal). In the long-term, you may set a goal to reduce your daily caloric intake to 2000 calories, consume at least 3-5 fruits and vegetables and give up butter for jelly. You can use Figure 9.3 to set your own SMAART goals to improve your nutritional habits.

S		
M		
A		
A		
R		
T		

Figure 9.3—Setting Nutritionally SMAART Goals

In addition to setting SMAART goals, you can also set Staircase goals to improve your nutritional habits just like those you created Chapters 6-8 (see Figure 9.4). In the situation described below, Shari never eats breakfast and she wants to start. On the bottom of the stairs, there is a zero for the number of times Shari presently eats breakfast. On the top of the stairs is Shari's long-term goal of eating breakfast seven days per week 17-18 weeks from now. Then on the first step up from the bottom is Shari's first short-term goal which is to have breakfast one time per week. So what are your short-term and long-term nutritional goals? Consider using the staircase. If it worked for Shari, it can work for you, too.

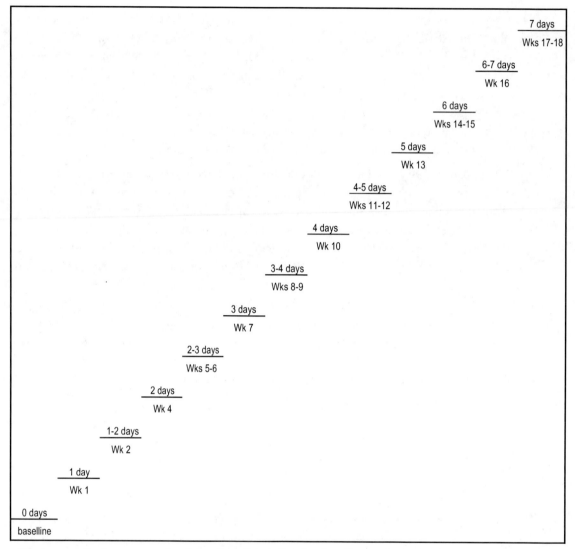

Shari presently does not eat breakfast (baseline = 0). Her first short-term goal is to eat breakfast 1 day per week and her long-term goal is to be eating breakfast seven days per week. Once Shari reaches her first short-term goal, she will set her next goal on the next step and so on. If at any time you do not reach your short-term goal, determine what stopped you and then incorporate the strategies you have learned to get back in action and climb the stairs toward your next goal.

Figure 9.4—Staircase Goals for Improving Nutritional Habits

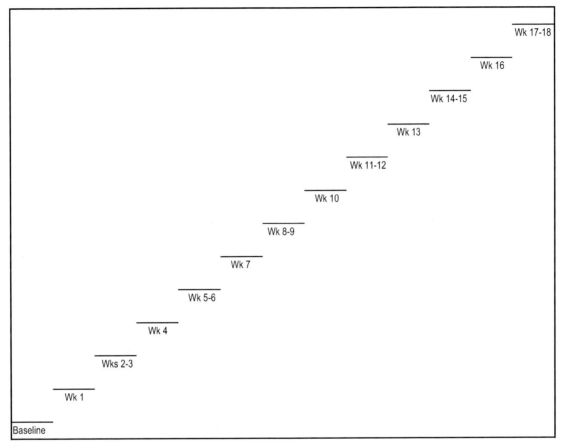

On the top of the stairs, put your long-term nutritional dream goal (e.g., eating fruits ___ times per day, drinking water ___ times per day, planning your meals ___ times per day). On the bottom of the stairs put your baseline and what you are presently doing. Then on the step just above your baseline, put your first short-term goal. Once you reach that goal, you can set a goal on the next step up and so on.

Figure 9.4—Staircase Goals for Improving Your Nutritional Habits

EVALUATING THE SUCCESS OF YOUR EATING HABITS

So, how successful were you? What changes did you make to your eating habits? Are you planning your meals more? Have you replaced unhealthy foods and beverages with healthy ones? Are you consuming more water? How conscious are you about what you eat? How much do you eat daily? Where do you eat? When do you eat?

Whatever your results were, praise yourself for the effort you put in. If you were indeed successful, then keep using the same strategies. Perhaps you are ready to make another change (e.g., replacing another unhealthy food with a healthy alternative, drinking one more glass of water per day). If you were not successful, then incorporate a different strategy. The important thing is to stay in action. Doing so will help you continue to take your commitment to eat and drink healthy into positive actions. Before you know it, you will have adopted a variety of strategies that work for you and positive nutritional habits will become a part of your everyday life.

REVIEW QUESTIONS

1. Explain five reasons why people eat poorly.

2. Define healthy eating.

3. Describe the differences between the old Food Guide Pyramid and the new Food Guide Pyramid.

4. Explain which pyramid you like better and why?

5. List the six essential nutrients and explain the functions of each.

6. Explain the difference between a macronutrient and a micronutrient.

7. Why is water the most important nutrient?

8. Approximately what percent of your diet should come from carbohydrates, fats and proteins?

9. How many calories are there in one gram of carbohydrates, fats, and proteins?

10. Define the components of an energy balance equation (EBE).

11. List five strategies that you can use to eat healthier. Which ones do you think will work for you and why?

12. How committed are you to use at least one or more of these strategies?

13. Explain the purposes of using SMAART goals to improve your nutritional habits. List at least one SMAART goal that you have to improve your present nutritional habits.

14. How will you determine the success of your eating habits?

LAB ASSIGNMENT 9.1
ANALYZING YOUR DIETARY CONSUMPTION

1. Using the dietary recall log in Appendix 9A, write down everything you eat and drink over a one week period. Include the type of food that you consumed and how it was prepared (e.g., raw, baked, grilled, fried) since that can effect the quality of the meal as well as total number of calories. Pay careful attention to the portion sizes that you intake since many times the portion size of the label is less than the portion size consumed. Consequently, you may be consuming more calories than you think. You can determine caloric intake by reading the nutrition labels of everything you consume as well as familiarizing yourself with a variety of nutritional information sources located in the reference section at the end of this chapter.

2. Under column 1 labeled "Meal" include the time that you had that particular meal.

3. Under the column 2 labeled "Planned/Spontaneous" determine if your meal was planned or spontaneous. A planned meal is a meal where you know what you are going to eat at least a few hours in advance. A spontaneous meal is defined as eating when you get hungry, not knowing in advance what you will eat

4. In column 3 labeled, "Length of time for meal" record how long each meal takes from the time you first started eating and drinking until your last bite and sip.

5. When the week is up, answer the following questions.

   a. How many calories did you consume each day?

Day 1	Day 2	Day 3	Day 4	Day 5	Day 6	Day 7

   b. When did you consume the majority of your calories?

   breakfast   lunch   dinner   snack

   c. How many calories did you consume for breakfast? lunch? dinner? snack?

Breakfast	Lunch	Dinner	Snack

   d. What percentage of your daily caloric intake came from carbohydrates, proteins, and fats?

   carbohydrates = _____ % + proteins = _____ % + fats = _____ % = 100%

e. Using the "Nutritional Awareness Chart," list all of the foods and beverages that are either too high in fat (over 30% of total calories comprised of fat; more than 20% total fat calories comprised of saturated fat), too high in simple sugars and/or have low or no nutritional value.

f. Rank each of the foods and beverages listed from question 5e on a scale of 1 (must have on a daily basis) to 9 (can do without) under the column listed unhealthy intake.

Nutritional Awareness Chart

Foods with over 30% of calories from fat	Foods & Drinks High in Simple Sugars	Foods & Drinks with little or no nutritional value	Ranking (1 must have it on a daily basis) to (9) I can do without it
			1 2 3 4 5 6 7 8 9
			1 2 3 4 5 6 7 8 9
			1 2 3 4 5 6 7 8 9
			1 2 3 4 5 6 7 8 9
			1 2 3 4 5 6 7 8 9
			1 2 3 4 5 6 7 8 9

g. Using the information listed above do you think you eat healthy? If so, explain why? If not, explain why not?

LAB ASSIGNMENT 9.2

1. Using the Healthy Alternative Chart, list the unhealthy foods or beverages that you have consumed over the past week and the frequency of times you had it. Then include a healthy alternative that you might consider to replace the unhealthy product (e.g., water for soda; jelly for butter, grilled chicken for fried chicken) over the next week.

Healthy Alternative Chart

Unhealthy Food or Beverage	Frequency of Times Consumed over the Past Week	Healthy Alternative

2. How committed are you to improving your nutritional habits and replacing at least one or more unhealthy food(s) and/or beverage(s) for healthy alternatives listed above?

So where are you on the commitment scale?

1	2	3	4	5	6	7

Not committed   Extremely committed

3. List 1-3 strategies that you will incorporate to improve your dietary habits this week?

_____

_____

_____

4. How motivated are you to incorporate these strategies into your nutritional plan this week?

So where are you on the commitment scale?

1	2	3	4	5	6	7

Not committed   Extremely committed

5. Are there anything stopping you from incorporating these new strategies? If so, list each and include a strategy to overcome these barriers.

6. After the week is up, evaluate the success of your eating habits.

   a. Did you adopt the healthy alternative(s) into your dietary habits this week? If so, how often and how do you feel about your accomplishment(s)? If not, explain why?

                         YES   NO

   b. How do you feel about your accomplishments?

   c. What do you have planned next week to improve your dietary habits?

REFERENCES AND RECOMMENDED READINGS

Bouchard, C., Bray, G.A., & Hubbard, V.S. (1990). "Basic and Clinical Aspects of Regional Fat Distribution. *American Journal of Clinical Nutrition*, 52, 946-950.

Duffy, R.L. (2002). ADA Complete Food and Nutrition Guide, 2nd ed. Chicago, IL: American Dietetic Association: An excellent review of current nutrition information.

Food and Nutrition Board, Institute of Medicine, 2002. *Dietary reference intakes for Energy, Carbohydrates, Fiber, Fat, Fatty Acids, Cholesterol, Protein, and Amino Acids.* Washington, D.C. National Academic Press.

FDA Center for Food Safety and Applied Nutrition. Provides information about topics such as food additives, food labels, and food borne illness.

U.S. Department of Health and Human Services, Department of Agriculture, *Nutrition and your health Dietary Guidelines for Americans,* Home and Garden Bulletin NP. 232 (Washington , DC:DHHS, 2000).

U.S. Department of Health and Human Services, Department of Agriculture, Center for Nutrition Policy and Information, 1996, Food Guide Pyramid, USDA Home and Garden Bulletin no. 252

Wilmore, J.H. (1994). Exercise and weight control: Myths, misconceptions, and quackery. ACSM, Indianapolis, IN, June 1994.

Wong, S.H.S., & Chung, S. (2003). Glycemic index: An educational tool for health and fitness professionals? *ACSM's Health and Fitness Journal*, November/December.

www.cdc.gov/nccdphp/dnpa/obesity = #1 reference cited...

www.cdc.gov guidelines/dga 2005 document

www.fitday.com

www.foodguidepyramid

www.health.gov/dietary guidelines/dga 2005 document

www.health.harvard.edu/press.

(www.usda.gov; www.uhealthcare.com/topics/weight/weightcontrol).

www.healthfitcounter.com

www.hhs.gov

(www.hsph.harvard.edu/nutrition source/pyramids.html)

www.my-calorie-counter.com

www.nutritionexplorations.org/educators/pyramid-main-asp

www.usda.gov.com

(www.usda.gov; www.uhealthcare.com/topics/weight/weightcontrol).

APPENDIX 9A

Meal	Planned or Spontaneous	Length of Time for Meal	What else were you doing besides eating?	Total Calories	Carb Cals	Fat Cals	Protein Cals
Breakfast							
Lunch							
Dinner							
Snack							

Chapter 10

Body Composition

OBJECTIVES

After reading this chapter, you will be able to:

- Define and assess body composition
- Distinguish among *underweight, overweight, overfat*, and *obese*
- Incorporate strategies to improve body composition
- Determine your level of commitment to improve body composition
- Recognize myths about improving your body composition

For many years, the traditional method of determining if you needed to gain or lose weight was to get on the scale to see how much you weighed and then compare your results with a standardized height-weight chart. If your weight exceeded the amount listed for your height, you were considered overweight and if your weight was below what was listed for your height, you were considered under weight.

Unfortunately, this method creates several problems. First, the scale only determines total body weight and not what your body weight consists of (e.g., muscle, bones essential and storage fat, etc). Second, the height/weight charts are based on norms or averages of weight and height; even though you may be above or below the average, you are not necessarily in an unhealthy range. Finally, scales do not distinguish overweight vs. overfat. For example, people who are muscularly fit and get on a scale may exceed their recommended weight because they have more muscle than the average person, and muscle weighs more than fat does. When determining whether you need to gain or lose weight, it is recommended that you should assess your body composition in conjunction with the scale. This will tell you what your total body weight consists of and help you decide if you need to lose or gain fat or muscle weight.

WHAT IS BODY COMPOSITION?

Body composition is an important component of health-related fitness. Having an optimal amount of body fat will help you to live healthier, have more energy, and feel better about yourself. It will also lower your risk of chronic diseases (e.g., heart disease, cancer, stroke, diabetes, obesity, high blood pressure) that are linked to excessive amounts of body fat. Body composition refers to what the body is made up of. It consists of lean body mass and total body fat. Lean body mass is composed of muscle, bones, organs and connective tissues. Body fat consists of two types: essential fat and storage fat. ***Essential fat*** is needed for normal bodily functions; it is found in muscle, nerves, bones, intestines, heart, liver, and lungs. ***Storage fat*** is the fat stored in adipose tissue, (just beneath the skin and around major organs in the body). This fat serves three basic functions:

1. as a secondary source of energy to be used during moderate to long bouts of exercise; stored fat allows you to exercise for long periods of time having consumed fewer calories than you expend in a given exercise period.)

2. as an insulator to retain body heat;

3. as a cushion to absorb physical trauma to the body—Imagine if you had the same amount of body fat around your heart, lungs, brain and other vital organs as you have around your knee cap. Even the slightest physical contact in any of these areas could result in serious injuries.

The amount of storage fat varies from person to person and is based on many factors including age, gender, heredity, diet, metabolism, and activity level. In general, excessive storage fat is usually the result of consuming more food and drink (input) than is used up (expended) from metabolic functions and physical activity (output). Essential fat consists of approximately 3% of the total weight in men and 12% of the total weight in women. Women have a higher percentage because part of their essential fat is sex-specific fat which is found in the breasts, uterus and other sex-related areas.

UNDERWEIGHT VS. OVERWEIGHT VS. OVER-FAT VS. OBESITY

Underweight refers to an extremely low body weight with a total percent body fat to be less than 8-12% for women and 3-5% for men. Underweight also refers to a body weight that is considered to be below the normal recommended weight for an individual's height, build and sex with a body mass index (BMI) of < 20 (www.wrongdiagnosis.com). While the prevalence of becoming underweight is less than becoming overweight or obese, having too little body fat can become dangerous and increase risks of certain illnesses including anemia, heart irregularities, osteoporosis, and anorexia nervosa www.wrongdiagnosis.com/u/underweight/

intro.htm). Some possible causes of becoming underweight are malnutrition, reduced or lost appetite, difficulty chewing, dental pain, excessive overtraining, digestive organ diseases, cancer, hyperthyrodiism, diabetes, and genetics).

Overweight is defined as having total body weight that exceeds the recommended range for good health. As alluded to earlier, being overweight often refers to exceeding the standard of recommended body weight based on actual height. It does not necessarily mean that you are too fat and need to lose weight. For example, if the recommended amount of weight for your height is 160 pounds and you exceed that by 10 pounds, it simply means that you weigh more than the average person who is your height. You are considered overweight and not necessarily overfat. In fact, there are many athletes who fall into this category (e.g., football players, body builders, wrestlers). Emmit Smith, the NFL's all time leading rusher is 5'10 and weighed 216 pounds at the height of his career. This weight is well over the recommended amount of weight for someone who is 5'10. However, if you were to examine the percentage of Mr. Smith's body fat, he would fall well within the recommended range, if not lower. The reason for Mr. Smith being overweight is his muscularity, not his amount of body fat.

Overfat refers to the condition of having too much body fat. According to experts, men should have about 12-18% fat, while women's should have about 18-22% fat. Interestingly, you can be overfat without being overweight. For example, if you body weight is considered appropriate for your height you would not be overweight. However, if your body fat exceeds 18% (if you are a man) or 22% (if you are a woman), then you would be considered overfat.

Obesity is defined as having an excessive amount of body fat with men being considered obese when they have at least 25% of their total body weight coming from fat while women are considered obese when their total body weight consists of at least 30% body fat. Obesity is a major concern for health in the United States because it raises the risk of heart disease, diabetes, some cancers, arthritis and other conditions.

Adult Obesity Rates Across the United States

Recent research has discovered an increase in the prevalence of adult obesity in the United States from 19.8% in 2000 to 32.2% in 2004 (Mokdad et al., 2003; Ogdan et al., 2006) to 33% in 2008. In 2008, only one state (Colorado) had a prevalence of obesity less than 20%. Thirty-two states had a prevalence equal to or greater than 25%; six of these states (Alabama, Mississippi, Oklahoma, South Carolina, Tennessee, and West Virginia) had a prevalence of obesity equal to or greater than 30% (www.rueters.com).

According to the American Obesity Association, about 25-30% of Americans (approximately 60 million) are obese and over 300,000 premature deaths occur each year from obesity, costing in excess of over $100 billion dollars annually and accounting for nearly 10 percent of the medical spending in the United States (AOA, 2007). This increase in obesity has continued since 1960 and while there has not been an increase in adult obesity in the last year, the numbers do not seem to be decreasing either.

Obesity in Children

Unfortunately, the increase in obesity over the last twenty to thirty years is not limited to adults. Obesity has now become more common in youngsters, too. Today's youth are considered the most inactive generation in history with approximately 30% of children (ages 6 to 11) overweight and over 15% obese. For adolescents (ages 12 to 19), about 30% are overweight with over 15 percent considered obese. (www.obesity.org/subs/fastfacts/obesity youth.shtml). This excess body fat found in childhood and adolescence has been linked to higher rates of overweight and obesity in adulthood resulting in increases in heart disease, stroke, and diabetes.

ASSESSING BODY COMPOSITION

Assessing body composition is a more accurate way of measuring percent body fat and determining if you need to lose, gain, or maintain present body weight than the bathroom scale. Three of the more popular methods used to assess body fat are: (1) underwater weighing; (2) bioelectrical impedence and (3) skinfold calipers. Each method will be defined and explained, but because the skinfold procedure is the most practical method across a variety of settings including at school, at home, at certain exercise facilities, and local youth centers, only procedures for using skinfold calipers will be presented.

Underwater weighing is considered the standard for assessing body composition and is considered the most accurate of all other body composition assessments. In this procedure, an individual is submerged and weighed underwater with his/her weight under water being compared to his/her weight outside of water. The percentages of fat and fat-free weight are calculated from body density. Since fat floats and muscle sinks, people with more body fat will weigh less under water while lean people will weigh more.

Strengths—Underwater weighing is a highly accurate method of assessing body composition.

Limitations—Underwater weighing requires the expertise of a well-trained technician who knows how to administer this assessment and analyze the data properly. The equipment needed can be quite expensive and the overall process is rather time consuming, thus limiting its practicality when used with large samples (e.g., exercise classes). In addition, not everyone feels comfortable in the water and may become anxious about the thought of being submerged under water.

Bioelectrical impedence—This technique determines percent body fat by placing electrodes on the body and measuring the resistance of a small amount of electrical current that runs through the body. Since lean tissue has more water around it than fat, it is a better conductor and less resistant to current than fat. Thus, the resistance to current for individuals with large amounts of body fat is greater because the adipose tissue (the fat that is just underneath the skin) has little water content and therefore is a poor conductor of electrical current.

Strengths: Bioelectrical impedence is fairly accurate and can be done quickly and relatively inexpensively.

Limitations: Individuals must avoid becoming overhydrated or underhydrated since the amount of water in the body can bias results. In addition, individuals may become anxious with the thought of allowing electrical current to run through their body.

Skinfold measurements—This procedure involves using calipers to measure the thickness of skinfolds at several different bodily sites. Some experts recommend measuring two to three sites (e.g., triceps-suprailium-thigh for women & chest-abdomen-thigh for men) and then incorporating the measurements into a formula to determine overall body fat. However, failure to measure skinfold at other sites (e.g., calf, back, triceps for men) will only increase the margin of error and make it difficult to accurately predict the amount of estimated body fat on an individual's entire body. Therefore, it is recommended that you should assess body fat on multiple sites throughout the body and use the actual measurements rather than a formula to determine actual body fat. This will reduce the margin of error and hopefully motivate you more to improve your body composition. (See Figure 10.1 to familiarize yourself with sites that can be used to assess body composition).

Strengths: Assessing body fat using skinfold calipers is a relatively simple procedure to implement and with a little practice it can be conducted properly. In addition, this procedure is inexpensive and it does not take a great deal of time to administer. Finally, it can be used in individual as well as small and large group settings including at home, school gymnasium or laboratory, local youth center and private and corporate exercise centers.

Limitations: There is an estimated margin of error of 3-4% when using a formula with limited sites measured. In addition, the margin of error can increase if test administrators do not have adequate experience using calipers and distinguishing between actual body fat and skin.

PROCEDURES FOR ASSESSING BODY FAT USING SKINFOLD CALIPERS

1. Consider using the following sites to measure body fat. For men, chest, abdomen, thigh, tricep, calf, back. For women, thigh, triceps, suprailium, calf, and back.
2. Using the thumb and index finger, gently grasp the thickness of each skin from each site
3. Place the caliper about ½ inch below your fingers and hold for three seconds.
4. Measure each site 3X and record to the nearest one-half millimeter.
5. Record the averages of the two closest readings.
6. Plan to measure each site every month and compare the actual results (measurements in millimeters) rather than a formula to estimate percent body fat. This will reduce the margin of error and more accurately determine improvement.

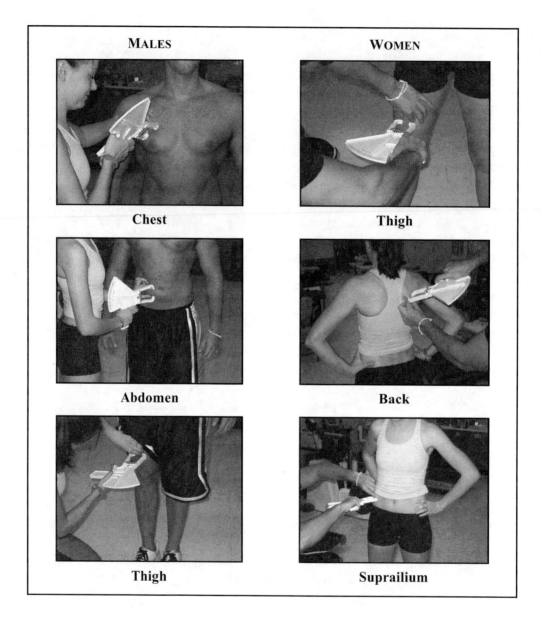

MALES

Chest

Abdomen

Thigh

WOMEN

Thigh

Back

Suprailium

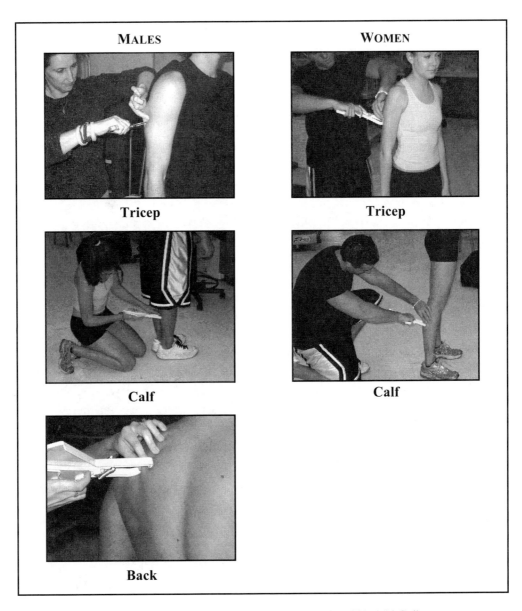

Figure 8.1—Assessing Body Composition Using Skinfold Calipers

IMPROVING YOUR BODY COMPOSITION

To improve your body composition, you should start off by being physically active and participating in cardiorespiratory, muscular fitness, and flexibility programs. Chapters 6-8 include health-related fitness programs designed specifically to meet your needs and match your level of commitment to be active in improving these areas. Next, focus on eating healthy, limiting foods high in saturated fat and incorporating the strategies identified in Chapter 9. Here are some strategies for you to consider when you want to change your body composition.

CHANGING YOUR BODY COMPOSITION

Losing Fat—If you want to lose fat, then you have to expend more energy than you consume. That means increasing your physical activity on a daily basis (e.g., walking instead of driving, taking the stairs instead of the elevator, exercising a few times per week) and eating properly. The goal is not only to lose fat weight, but to keep it off. As long as you continue to stay physically active and eat healthy, then losing fat weight and keeping it off will become a realistic goal.

Gaining Weight—If you want to gain weight, you have two choices: (1) eat more calories than you expend or (2) build muscle. If you plan on eating more calories, make sure that your percent body fat is below the recommended amount (10-12% for women and 5-8% for men) and focus on eating more from the new Food Guide Pyramid (www.mypyramid.gov) presented in Chapter 9. If you want to build muscle in order to gain weight then you need to work more on strengthening your muscles to give you the added weight you desire. That means working out with a higher weight (at least 70%-90% of your one-rep max).

Although many people choose to exercise in order to lose weight, it is important to remember that this may not be a realistic goal. As you get older your metabolism will naturally slow down and losing weight becomes more difficult. Therefore, your focus should be on being more physically active and eating healthy. Doing so will make you feel better and thus help to you see all the physical improvements that are certain to occur from participating in this type of lifestyle.

DETERMINING YOUR COMMITMENT TO HAVE A HEALTHY BODY COMPOSITION

On a scale of 1-9 (check commitment scale), circle your level of commitment towards having a healthy body composition.

           1   2   3   4   5   6   7   8   9
    Low commitment   **Moderate Commitment**   **High Commitment**

If you selected anything less than 7, then there is probably something stopping you from making a full commitment. Therefore, you should identify what those barriers might be and use some of the strategies discussed in Ch 9 to improve your eating habits, design an exercise program that fits into your life (Chapters 6-8) and set SMAART goals (Chapter 3) that motivate you to have fun and improve your health-related fitness.

Recognizing Myths about How to Improve Body Composition

There are many myths about how to lose fat and tone muscles with minimum or no work involved. Unfortunately, some people believe these myths and become disheartened when the claims made about the product or method proves to be false. Here are a few of the more popular myths about exercise and body composition followed by a realistic explanation of what you can do to achieve your health-related fitness goals.

1. ***Doing abdominal work like sit ups turns stomach fat into muscle*** —Wouldn't it be great if you do a few reps of sit ups and turn that unwanted stomach fat into washboard abs? This procedure is more commonly known as "Spot Reducing" which is based on the belief that you can reduce body fat from designated places on the body. Unfortunately, this is not possible for several reasons. First, you cannot turn fat into muscle. Fat is fat and muscle is muscle. In order to see toned muscles, you have to get rid of the fat and that happens from eating properly and working on your cardiovascular endurance and muscular fitness. Second, there is no exercise that guarantees you will lose fat from a certain area on your body. Just like when you overeat, you do not know exactly where the body fat will be stored. When you exercise, you cannot accurately assume that fat as energy will come only from the place(s) that you want. However, the tendency is that if you have an area of your body where you tend to have a higher portion of body fat, there is a good chance that when your energy expenditure exceeds your energy input, some of the fat that is used for energy will come from that area.

   Reality: What you need to do! First, eat healthy and make sure you do not overeat. Next, increase your CRE by exercising for longer amounts of time each week. This will help you expend more and more calories. Finally, work on toning your major muscle groups. This will make your body look better and increase your metabolism which will help to expend more calories at rest.

2. ***Skipping meals helps me lose weight***—That could be true. If you skip meals and are consuming fewer calories in a day than you expend then you will lose weight. However, if you are not physically active and you are losing in excess of two or more pounds per week, then the weight you are losing is most probably coming from water, not fat. In time, you will have to replace the water or you will become dehydrated. It is also important to point out that skipping meals does not guarantee that you will lose weight, especially if you overeat during your other meals or consume a significant portion of your caloric intake later in the day and evening. If you are physically active and exercise and you skip meals then the quality of your workouts will decrease. Over time, you will not have enough energy in your body to help you over-

load during your workouts and thus your physical improvements (e.g., exercising for longer amounts of time, increasing intensity) will diminish.

Reality: What you need to do—Rather than skipping meals, eat the right foods in smaller portions. This will give you more energy to be more physically active throughout the day which can result in a greater expenditure of caloric output and help you to get rid of excessive body fat.

3. ***Lifting weights creates big muscles for women***—While there are some women that train competitively for body building and power lifting and have developed large muscles, it is important to note that these women train significantly harder and put significantly more time and effort into their workouts than is recommended for most women who simply want to get fit and stay fit and improve their physical appearance by toning their muscles. In addition, it is important for you to know that women do not have enough of the male hormone, testosterone to allow for producing large muscle growth.

Reality: What you need to do! Women should give weight training a try by working on the major muscle groups a few times per week. All you need to do is choose 2-3 exercises per body part and perform 1-2 sets per exercise lifting approximately 50-60% of your max or (12-15 reps per set). This regimen will help women to tone and define their muscles, not make them grow large. See Chapter 7 for a list of possible muscular fitness programs designed specifically for you.

4. ***Eating more protein will get me bigger muscles and improve my health***—While protein does serve a role in repairing muscle tissue, eating too much of it will not create bigger muscles unless you work on improving your muscular strength. In fact, according to medical experts, a diet in which protein makes up more than 30% of your daily caloric intake could cause more harm than good. As your caloric intake of protein increases over 30% it causes a buildup of toxic ketones which can overwork kidneys by having to flush these ketones from your body. As your kidneys rid your body of these toxic ketones, you can lose a significant amount of water, which puts you at risk of dehydration, particularly if you exercise heavily (Butterfield as cited by Cole-Peralta, (2007) & Nelson, 2002).

Another problem with excessive protein intake is that it can increase storage fat build up and thus increase risk of coronary heart disease. Finally, if you increase protein intake and deplete yourself of complex carbohydrates you can overwork the dietary system and increase the risk of illness. For more information on the risks of consuming too much protein please read Cousens, G atwww.creationsmagazine. com/articles/c108/counsens.html.

Reality: Stick to eating a well balanced diet. This will give your body as much protein as it needs to perform the role that it is meant to (approximately 15-25% of your caloric intake). If you want bigger muscles then work on improving your muscular strength by lifting 70% or more of your max and performing 2-8 reps per set.

5. *No pain, no gain!* Some people think that in order to improve the way their body looks they must feel pain during their workouts. Thankfully, this is not true. You do not need to nor should you want to feel pain during exercise. In fact, feeling pain may be a sign that you are overdoing it and at risk of injury.

    Reality: Overload your body so that you feel tension, not pain. Recognize the signs and systems of overloading each system during workouts. For example, know what your heart rate should be during aerobic activity. You should always be able to talk and you should never be out of breath. During muscular fitness training, you should feel tension in the working muscles during lifting that eases up in between sets. Finally, during flexibility exercises, you should feel tension while stretching that decreases in intensity the longer the stretch is held for. Once you recognize how to create tension rather than pain, you will see that there are enormous gains without pain!

6. *Being skinny means you are physically fit*—Having a low percent body fat or looking thin does not necessarily mean you are physically fit especially if you became thin only from dieting and you are not physically active. Through dieting, you have addressed one important component of health-related fitness (body composition), however, you may have neglected the other important components (cardiorespiratory endurance, muscular fitness, flexibility).

    Reality: Focus more on being physically fit by exercising regularly and overloading the components of health-related fitness such as cardiorespiratory endurance, muscular fitness, flexibility, and eating healthy. Then if you become skinny, it will be for the right reasons.

7. *Muscle turns to fat when you stop exercising*—Although it is common to gain weight when you stop exercising for extended periods of time, it is not because the muscle has turned to fat. When muscles are not being overloaded or when they are used in a reduced capacity, they can lose size as well as shape. If you start overeating you will increase the amount of stored fat, resulting in what looks like fat replacing muscle.

    Reality: Once again, stay physically active and eat healthy. In times when you are not able to stick to your exercise program, work on being as physically active as possible (e.g., walking instead of driving to local places, doing a few toning exercises before going to bed). Plan to get at least one workout in per week during this time period in order to maintain your present level of fitness. Avoid overeating especially now that you have reduced your exercising frequency and time. Most important, work on a new plan of action that helps you to fit exercise back into your life.

In conclusion, you now know what body composition is and how to assess your own body composition to determine if you are in a healthy range. You have been introduced to the myths about how to improve body composition, as well as being given some real strategies for improving body composition. Remember the old phrase, "You are what you eat!" Well, if you want to be look fit, be physically fit and most important live a healthy lifestyle then you have to make sure that you eat healthy and exercise properly.

REVIEW QUESTIONS

1. What is the problem with using height/weight charts to determine if you need to lose or gain weight?

2. Define body composition.

3. What is the difference between essential fat and storage fat?

4. What are the three roles that fat plays in the body?

5. Describe the differences between someone who is overfat from someone who is overweight?

6. Define obesity and explain what can be done to avoid being obese?

7. Name three ways you can assess body composition and explain the strengths and limitations of each approach.

8. Which body composition technique do you like most, least, and why?

9. Discuss the procedure for assessing body composition using skinfold calipers.

10. Explain why you are better off using actual measurements rather than a formula to determine actual body composition.

11. What suggestions can you offer someone who wanted to improve his/her body composition?

12. List at least two strategies that you will consider using to maximize your commitment to have a healthy body composition.

13. List at least three myths about how to improve body composition.

14. What suggestions can you offer someone who believes in these myths?

Lab Assignment 10.1

Your assignment is to find an advertisement via the internet, newspaper, magazine, commercial, or infomercial on any of the following topics: (1) losing body weight; (2) turning body fat into muscle; (3) diets; (4) nutritional supplements; (5) exercise equipment that promotes significant changes in the body;

1. Determine how accurate the information being presented is?

2. Is the information being advertised consistent with the research. Please be sure to cite research to support your position.

3. If you were to conduct your own infomercial on body composition, list five important facts that you would like to communicate to your audience.

4. Explain three strategies that you would recommend to help people obtain the proper percent of body fat.

5. Describe the proper method for using skinfold calipers.

References and Recommended Readings

American Dietetic Association www.eatright.org

American Obesity Association (2006). www.obesity.org

Bray, G. (1993). The nutrient balance approach to obesity. Nutrition Today, 28, 13-18.

Clark, N. (1991). How to gain weight healthfully. *Physician and Ssportsmedicine* 19, 53.

Clarkson, P.M. (1998). The skinny on weight loss supplements and drugs: Winning the war against fat. *ACSM's Health and Fitness Journal*: 18

Counsens, G. www.creationsmagazine.com/articles/c108/counsens.html.

Hedley, A.A., Ogden, C.L., Johnson, C.L., Carroll, M.D., Curtin, L.R., & Flegal, K.M. (2004). Prevalence of overweight and obesity among US children, adolescents, and adults, 1999-2002. *Journal of the American Medical Association*, 292: 2847-2850.

Kassirer, J.P., & Angell, M. (1998). Losing weight-An il-fated new year's resolution. *New England Journal of Medicine*, 338, 52-54.

Klarenbach, S., Padwal, R., Chuck, A., & Jacobs, P. (2006). Population-based analysis of obesity and workforce participation. *Obesity*, 14, 920-927.

Lichtenstein, A.H., Appel, L.J., Brands, M., Carnethon, M., Daniels, S., Franch, H.A., Franklin, B., Kris-Etherton, P., Harris, W.S., Howards, B., Karanja, N., Lefevre, M.,

Rudel, L., Sacks, F., Van Horn, L., Winston, M., & Wylie-Rosett, J. (2006). Diet and lifestyle recommendations revision 2006. A scientific study from the American Heart Association Nutrition Committee, Circulation, 114, 82-96.

Mokdad, A.H., Ford, E.S., Bowman, B.A., Dietz, W.H., Vinicor, F., Bales, V.S., & Marks, J.S. (2003). Prevalence of obesity, diabetes, and obesity-related health risk factors. *Journal of the American Medical Association,* 289,76-79.

Nelson, M. (2202). Will eating more protein help your body gain muscle? www.medicine.-net.com

Ogden, C.L., Carroll, M.D., Curtin, L.R., McDowell, M.A., Tabak, C. J. Tabak, Flegal, K.M. (2006). Prevalence of overweight and obesity in the United States, 1999-2004. *Journal of the American Medical Association, 295,* 1549-1555.

Pardo Silva, M.C., De Laet, C., Nusselder, W.J., Mamum, A.A. & Peeters, A. (2006). Adult obesity and the number of years lived with and without cardiovascular disease. *Obesity,* 14, 1264-1273.

Peralta, K.C. (2007). How much protein should you eat? www.americanchronicle.com/-articles/view/Article.asp?articleID=25079

www.mypyramid.gov

www.obesity.org/subs/fastfacts/obesityyouth.shtml)

www.rueters.com

Chapter 11

Cognitive Strategies: Learning How and What to Think During Exercise

OBJECTIVES

After reading this chapter, you will be able to:

- Define cognitive strategies
- Incorporate association, dissociation, positive self-talk and imagery into your exercise program
- Evaluate the effectiveness of using cognitive strategies to enhance your exercise enjoyment, motivation, and performance
- Determine your level of commitment to use different cognitive strategies during exercise

An important part of your exercise program involves your thoughts or cognitions—what you focus your attention on during exercise (Weinberg & Gould, 2003). If you find exercise boring and difficult, then you probably will lose your interest and your incentive to continue will diminish. But, if you like what you are doing and your mind is filled with positive thoughts during exercise, you enjoy it more and become more inclined to find time to fit it into your life.

One of the most popular reasons for not exercising is because it is perceived to be boring. Whether the feeling of boredom is related to the activity itself (e.g., doing the same thing over and over), the environment it is in (being in the same place and not liking the surroundings, e.g., dark, cold, old equipment), the people around you (feeling uncomfortable, not perceiving that you have anything in common with those around you, focusing on differences more than similarities), many people stop exercising because they do not like it and it is boring to them.

In this chapter, you will learn what cognitive strategies are and how to incorporate them into your exercise program in order to create an empowering atmosphere that will increase your enjoyment and desire to make exercise an integral part of your life. So rather than wish exercise was more enjoyable, now you can plan to make it happen!

WHAT ARE COGNITIVE STRATEGIES?

Cognitive strategies are structured ways of thinking: they are designed to enhance performance and/or enjoyment in exercise and sport. In essence, cognitive strategies are ways to program your thoughts. The following section introduces two different cognitive strategies, (association and dissociation) and it describes how you can use each to maximize enjoyment, productivity and safety during your exercise workouts. The thinking starts now!

Association is defined as concentrating on the relevant or related aspects of the activity or exercise (e.g., how the muscles feel, breathing rate, pacing, technique) for which you are engaged in. For example, if you are going for a run, associating would involve focusing on important factors related to running (e.g., heart rate, breathing pattern, pace, form, muscular tension, how your body feels, how much energy you believe you have in order to complete the desired distance or time). If you are working on muscular fitness, association would involve concentrating on proper form, correct breathing, how your muscles feel from one rep to the next and knowing how much strength it will take to complete a given set. Finally, associating while working on flexibility would involve concentrating on proper form, on identifying and stretching to your tension point, and on making sure your body is in the correct position and knowing when to stretch a little further.

Dissociation is defined as concentrating on the irrelevant or unrelated aspects of the activity or exercise for which you are engaged in. Dissociation is designed to take your mind off of exercise and onto things that you enjoy, thus enhancing your overall exercise experience. For example, dissociation while exercising may include listening to music while going for a run, watching television while stretching, reading in between sets of lifting weights, and talking with an exercise partner during CRE, MF or flexibility activities. With each strategy, your focus centers on engaging your mind with information unrelated to exercise.

The challenge is knowing when to associate or dissociate during exercise. Three factors to consider when deciding whether you should adopt associative or dissociative strategies during exercise are safety, performance, and enjoyment.

Safety—For individuals who are starting out and first getting accustomed to the demands of the exercise, association should be the cognitive strategy used. By listening to your body and focusing on using proper technique, determining the right pace and knowing how and when to increase or decrease the time and intensity, you will decrease your chances of injury, prevent undo fatigue, and ultimately increase your performance/fitness level.

Performance—According to research, association has been found to increase performance more than dissociation during competitive running (Morgan & Pollack, 1977; Masters & Olges, 1988; Nietfeld, 2003), swimming (Couture, Jerome, & Tihanyi, 1999), and rowing (Scott, Scott, Bedic, & Dowd, 1999*)*. If you are primarily motivated to improve your exercise performance (e.g., run faster, stretch further, lift more) you should associate by concentrating on the demands of the exercise and how your body is adapting to it. For example, when running, you should know when to conserve your energy and when you need to pick up the pace. When lifting weights, you should know how many reps you plan to achieve and how much strength it will take to get it done. Finally, for flexibility, you should know where you tension point is and concentrate on holding the stretch for a prescribed amount of time that will improve your range of motion in the desired area(s). So if you want to increase your performance then think about what you are doing.

Enjoyment—One of the most effective ways to increase your enjoyment is to combine exercise with other activities that you like to do. For example, listening to your favorite music while you go for your walk, run, or bike ride, reading an interesting book while riding your stationary bicycle, or working out with a friend and engaging in a friendly conversation can all take your mind off of your exercise activity and onto something with a greater perceived enjoyment. Interestingly, research has found that dissociation has been favored during practice or recreational activity and has led to higher levels of exercise enjoyment, better attendance and greater compliance of exercise than association (Martin, et al., 1984). In other words, because you are focusing on things that stimulate you, you pay less attention to some of the things you may not like while exercising (repetitiveness, fatigue, muscular tension, unappealing location).

INCORPORATING ASSOCIATION AND DISSOCIATION INTO YOUR EXERCISE PROGRAM

Association

Association should be used when you are familiarizing yourself with an activity or exercise and you need to learn and/or focus on the proper form and technique (e.g., bodily position), the demands of the exercise (e.g., muscular tension, heart rate, pace) and how your body responds to these demands (e.g., fatigue, feeling energized). For example, when you first begin to exercise, you should focus on making sure you are doing the exercise properly and pay attention to how your body feels. Are you comfortable? If you are using equipment like a bicycle, are you seated in the correct position? If you are on a treadmill, are you going at the right pace? How do your legs feel? How is your breathing? If you are lifting weights, are you sitting or standing properly? Is your body weight centered? Is the fulcrum range of motion lever inserted in the correct position, creating the proper range of motion? When stretching, are you properly warmed up? Is your body in the correct position for each stretch? What is your tension point and how long do you plan on holding a stretch for?

Associating During CRE Activity

Here is a list of guidelines used to determine when and how to associate during CRE activity.

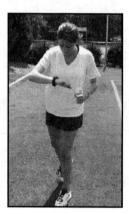

1. ***Familiarize yourself with the demands of the activity*** (e.g. using correct form; using equipment properly; taking the correct position; learning the proper pace for your current level of fitness; checking your heart rate)

2. ***Make sure your body is warmed up and ready***—Listen to your body to determine when you are warmed up and ready to begin exercise overload.

3. ***Set the right pace***—Start off going slow and think about how your body feels. Pay specific attention to how you are breathing and the muscular tension you are experiencing, particularly in the lower extremities (quadriceps, hamstring, calves, hip flexors, ankles).

4. ***Making sure your heart rate is in the correct zone***—Every few minutes, you should monitor your heart rate to make sure that you are working at the right intensity. If your heart rate is too high (above your training zone) you will be breathing heavily and need to slow down and if your heart rate is too low (below your training zone) the exercise will feel too easy and then you can speed up.

5. ***Identifying how much energy you have***—At the start of your workout as well as every few minutes during your exercise, you should check in with yourself and determine how much energy you have. You always want to feel like your perceived amount of energy can match or exceed the energy demands of your activity. This way you will feel more comfortable during exercise and increase your time/duration or intensity if you so desire. If the energy demands of the activity are greater than your perceived amount of energy, then you know it is time to slow down and/or stop.

6. ***To increase performance***—If your primary goal is to increase your CRE performance (e.g., training for races or competition), association can help you to focus on pacing yourself, knowing when to conserve (slow down) and expend energy (pick up the pace), maximize proper form and control your breathing.

Dissociating During CRE Activity

With CRE activity, the exercises you perform are rhythmic in nature and generally can be learned within a short period of time. Once you learn the proper form and pace, you can begin to dissociate if you like. In fact, you will probably enjoy your CRE exercises more when you dissociate since you will be able to decide what you want to think about rather than focusing on how much longer you have to go or how bored you are.

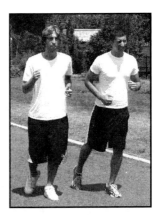

1. *Know What & How to Do*—Once you become familiar with the types of exercise you want to do and you know how to do them properly, you can plan to incorporate other activities that your enjoy and take your mind off of exercise (e.g., listening to music, talking with a friend, watching TV, texting).

2. *Feel Comfortable*—Once you feel comfortable during your aerobic activities and you no longer have to think about what to do (e.g., pacing and proper form are automatic), you can incorporate dissociation into your workout.

3. *Replace Boredom for Fun*—If you find your workouts boring and monotonous and you have lost your desire to exercise on a regular basis, the time has come to make things more fun. Listed below are several dissociative strategies to consider.

- Listen to music
- Exercise with a friend
- Read
- Watch TV
- Play a video game
- Use the time to plan your day on your PDA
- Talk on the telephone.
- Text Messages
- Surf the Net or Email on your I-phone

Associating during Muscular Fitness Training

Associating is a very important technique when working on muscular fitness. The intensity of this type of training is greater than CRE or flexibility exercise and as a result there is

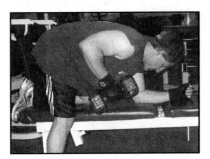

greater risk of injury. Therefore, it is important for you to know what to focus on (e.g., concentrating on the correct form, choosing the correct weight, controlling and balancing the weight properly, breathing properly, knowing how many reps you will to do, etc.). Here are some guidelines for how and when to associate during muscular fitness training.

Warming Up—If you are working on a new body part or beginning a new exercise, you should begin with a warm up, using a light weight for approximately 8-12 reps. During this time, you should be concentrating on how your body feels as you prepare yourself for exercise overload.

Using Correct Form—Each exercise that you do requires you to use the correct form-- starting at the correct position, knowing how to lift the weight properly, using your full range of motion, and controlling the weight on the exertion (lifting) and resting (put the weight back to the stack or initial starting place) phases.

Listening to your body—While lifting, you need to know what your body is capable of doing and not doing. Listening to your body can help you recognize when you might be able to do a few more reps, as well as when you are at your limit and need to stop.

Lifting to the Full Range of Motion—Each exercise that you do requires that your lift goes to the full range of motion. That means that you should be concentrating on fully extending and contracting on every repetition. When using machines, you must know where to place the fulcrum (the knob that determines range of motion).

Counting Your Reps– Each repetition should take between 3 and 5 seconds to complete. One to 2 seconds should be devoted to the exertion phase (lifting the weight) and 3-4 seconds should be devoted to the resting phase (bringing the weight back to its' initial starting point). Concentrating on counting how long each phase of each rep will take will help you to properly overload your muscles and get a better workout.

Once you finish your set, you should evaluate how your body feels. Are your muscles feeling tight, sore, and fatigued, or are you invigorated and strong? Concentrating on how your muscles feel will provide you with important information about how you will proceed with the rest of your workout. For example, if you feel tired, but want to continue, you may need to more time to rest in between sets, reduce the weight on the next set of the same exercise, or select a different exercise or body part to work on next. Conversely, if you think you can do more, then you may decide that increasing the weight on the next set will give you a better workout.

Dissociating During Muscular Fitness Training

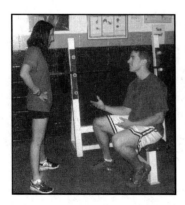

The only time you should be dissociating during muscular fitness training is in between sets or exercises. It is simply too dangerous and unsafe to take your mind off of what you are doing while working on your muscular fitness. However, once you have become used to how your body feels and you are familiar with the demands of your workouts, you can begin to dissociate in between sets by listening to music, reading, talking to someone in between sets or using a journal to write down any thoughts that may enter your mind. Just remember that once your rest time has been completed, it is time to associate and begin concentrating on your next set.

Associating During Flexibility Training

The same rules apply for using association and dissociation during flexibility training as for CRE & MFT. First, you have to know how to stretch safely and then you should always start off associating to make sure your body is ready to be stretched. Are you warmed up before your stretch? Are your muscles ready to be stretched? Concentrate on identifying and stretching to your tension point. Once you are there, then you have the following choices: (1) continue associating by focusing on the tension that you are feeling and striving to achieve a new tension point (seeing if you can stretch further over time); (2) breath rhythmically by inhaling while stretching to your tension point and exhaling to relax yourself while stretching or (3) focusing on achieving a new tension point by reaching just a little bit further.

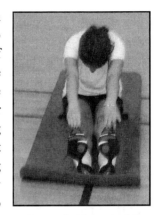

Dissociating During Flexibility Exercise

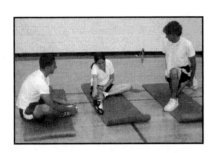

Once you have learned the correct way to perform your flexibility exercises and you have identified your proper tension point you can now begin to take your mind off of the common discomfort of stretching and dissociate. Here are a few ideas of how and when to dissociate during flexibility training.

Listen to Music—Some people find stretching boring and a perfect way to spice up your flexibility program is with a little music that makes you feel good. Simply put the music on in the background to establish an environment that creates a positive, yet relaxing mood state.

Stretch with a Partner—Stretching with a partner can help you to take your mind off of any negative thoughts about stretching and onto more pleasant thoughts. For example, if you and your partner are competitive and enjoy challenging one another, you can make stretching into a friendly competition by seeing who can stretch farther and longer. Perhaps, you have difficulty reaching your tension point by yourself or holding your stretch for more than a few seconds. Incorporating the use of a partner and having him/her talk to you while stretching may help you redirect your thoughts from associating on physical stress to dissociating with your partner.

Watching Television—An excellent way to dissociate while stretching is to watch television during certain parts of the show (e.g., commercials, first five minutes) and take your mind off how your body feels. After a few minutes, your body should feel better and help you to stretch for longer periods of time.

The way you communicate with yourself prior to, during, and after exercise can have a huge influence on how well you perform and how much you enjoy exercise. For example, if you talk negatively to yourself about exercise (e.g., "I don't like this"; "I will never see results," "This is so boring"), it is likely that in time you will somehow find a "reason" not to exercise. After all, why would you want to find the time to exercise when you are thinking negatively about it? However, if you talk positively to yourself about exercise, you will be more motivated to do it, perform at a higher level and get more out of it. The following section focuses on how to use cognitive strategy #3, *"Positive Self-Talk"* in your exercise program.

POSITIVE SELF-TALK

Positive self-talk is an internal dialogue that emphasizes increasing energy, effort and positive attitude (Weinberg & Gould, 2003). Positive self talk has been used to enhance performance, concentration, motivation, confidence, learning new skills, breaking bad habits, initiating action and sustaining effort.

According to Mikes (1987) 6 rules for creating self-talk should be used:

1. keep your phrases short and specific
2. use the first person and the present tense
3. construct positive phrases
4. say your phrases with meaning and intention
5. speak kindly to yourself
6. repeat phrases often

An example of how to use these six rules during exercises is listed below:

"I can do it!" is a short and specific phrase that can have a powerful effect. Using "I" brings the focus only on oneself. The phrase is positive since it emphasizes what you want to accomplish. There is meaning in the phrase, and the intention is to complete whatever workout you are committed to doing. Believing that you can do it is certainly being kind to yourself, and each time you are faced with uncertainty or doubt, stating "I can do it," "I can do it," "I can do it" will replace any negative thoughts with positive thoughts and keep you focused on succeeding rather than giving up! So what positive phrase(s) do you have that will increase your exercise performance, enjoyment and commitment?

Related to positive self-talk is a technique called *Thought Stopping*. Thought stopping is a process whereby you identify negative thoughts and then use a cue or trigger to stop the thought and clear your mind. For example, how often have you started exercising and discovered your mind was filled with negative thoughts like, "I don't want to do this right now," "I'm not in the mood to exercise," This is boring," only to feel guilty and upset later in the day if you allowed these negative thoughts to stop you from exercising.

Transforming Negative Self-Talk to Positive Self-Talk

The first step towards transforming negative thoughts into positive thoughts is to recognize that you are talking or thinking negatively to yourself. The next step is to use a cue word or phrase like "Stop" "Move on" or "Keep Going." You can also use a trigger, a quick gesture like clapping your hands, snapping your fingers, or tapping your thigh. The cue helps to stop the negative thoughts. The final step is to select a positive cue or phrase that will redirect your thoughts and energy onto what you want to accomplish while exercising.

While it is certainly common for people to have negative thoughts about exercising either before (e.g., I don't feel like exercising today, I'm not in the mood to exercise) or during exercise (this is boring, I don't want to keep going, I'm tired), recognizing negative thought patterns and immediately putting a stop to them and then transforming the negative into positive self-statements is a powerful way to increase productivity and enjoyment. Table 11.1 displays an example of how to transform negative thoughts into positive thoughts. Using Appendix 11A, your assignment now is to list any negative thoughts that you may have about exercise in the left hand column and in the right hand column list a cue word or phrase that transforms your negative self-talk into positive self-talk.

Table 11.1
Transforming Negative Self-Talk Into Positive Self-Talk
(This is an example for the students)

I'm too tired to exercise today	Exercise will energize me!
Exercise is boring	Exercise is exciting!
I don't have time to exercise today	Exercise will create more time for me to get things done!
Stop and do it later	Now it is best time!
I'll never see results	I am feeling better already!
I hate working out in this place	I choose my work out sites!
It's not fair that I have to do this	I want to do this!
I'll never be as fit as I used to be	I'm in better shape today than yesterday!
It's not working	I will make it work!

USING IMAGERY WITH EXERCISE

The fourth and final cognitive strategy for you to use with exercise is called ***Imagery***. Imagery is defined as creating or recreating an experience in the mind through the use of the senses (Vealy & Greenleaf, 2006). It is a mental training technique that teaches the mind to respond as programmed. You can use imagery before, during and after exercise in any of the following ways: (1) to prepare yourself to get ready for exercise; (2) help yourself focus on exercising properly and enjoying what you are doing; (3) to accomplish challenging goals and increase performance; (4) to feel your body become energized; (5) to overcome fatigue and persevere through your workout in order to achieve new performance levels (e.g., finishing that 10K race, getting that extra set in, stretching further than you ever have before and holding longer, too) and (6) to evaluate the success of your workout and correct any mistakes made so future workouts can become more efficient. For example, imagine if you took a few minutes out of your busy day to image how great you would feel later in the day after a workout. You begin to feel invigorated as you see yourself getting a good workout and think about the new performance levels that you have reached (e.g., reaching a new tension point, achieving a new level on the exercise bike, going for your longest run, getting in that extra rep on the chest press). Before you know it, you start to feel better about yourself and probably look forward to finishing up school or work and getting to the gym to exercise.

Using imagery effectively with exercise takes a little practice. There are three elements of good imagery: (1) Vividness, the clarity of the image; (2) Controllability, your ability to hold the desired image without distraction; and (3) Sensory Awareness, the ability to utilize the senses to create a realistic sensory experience.

So take a few minutes and image your next workout. Imagine that you are exercising in a place that is aesthetically pleasing and enjoyable. Imagine the exercises that you plan to do, and imagine achieving your desired exercise goals. Imagine feeling energized all throughout the workout and being in a positive mood. Through the use of imagery you will learn to create powerfully positive experiences with exercising, thus increasing your motivation and commitment to keep exercise in your life. Here are some suggestions for how to use imagery prior to, during and after exercise.

Using Imagery Before Exercise

Select a time anywhere between a few minutes and a few hours before your planned workout and image that you are going to have your best workout ever. See yourself improving your performance by exercising longer and challenging yourself to reach new levels of fitness. Envision an environment in which you like to exercise (e.g., exercise facility, at home, workplace). Hear the sounds of your favorite music. Feel how your body becomes invigorated with each rep, set, and minute that you exercise.

Using Imagery During Exercise

While exercising, you can use imagery to create experiences that help you enjoy your workouts, improve performance and increase your motivation to continue. For example, you can image running on the beach while on a treadmill. You can image yourself looking and feeling great after performing a new exercise or getting in a few extra reps. You can image yourself stretching to a new tension point and feeling more flexible than ever. By creating an image of what you want to accomplish and using your senses to make it seem real, you are using your mind to prepare your body to achieve new performance levels.

Using Imagery After Exercise

After finishing your workout, you can use imagery as part of your cool-down period. You can imagine the tension caused from exercise overload disappearing and being replaced with a huge sense of accomplishment. You can imagine feeling energized as you think about how much better you feel after your workout than before you started. You can imagine hearing people compliment you on how good you look and you can imagine seeing yourself in the best shape of your life.

DETERMINING YOUR LEVEL OF COMMITMENT TO INCORPORATE COGNITIVE STRATEGIES INTO YOUR EXERCISE PROGRAMS

Use the scale below to determine how committed you are to use one or more of the four cognitive strategies (association, dissociation, positive self-talk, and imagery) to enhance exercise enjoyment and performance. On a scale of 1-9, circle your level of commitment to use at least one or more cognitive strategy with exercise.

1   2   3   4   5   6   7   8   9

Not Committed   **Extremely Committed**

If for any reason you are not "extremely committed" to using cognitive strategies during exercise, take a few moments and write down what is stopping you. Then proceed to the next section with an open mind and by the time you are finished you will truly embrace the value of knowing how and what to think about during exercise.

Using Cognitive Strategies During Exercise

The goal of this chapter is to show how valuable cognitive strategies can be to increasing performance, enjoyment, motivation, and commitment to exercise. Whether it is using **association** to make sure you exercise safely and concentrate on incorporating proper technique; **dissociation** to take your mind off the demands of exercise and direct it to pleasing thoughts); **positive self-talk** to communicate the benefits that you are getting through exercise; or **imagery** to create an experience that prepares you to exercise, helps you during exercise, or allows you to evaluate your workouts positively after exercise, cognitive strategies are an excellent way to program your thoughts to work for you with exercise. You can determine which one(s) are for you as you practice each of these strategies in your lab assignments. Enjoy and think positively!

REVIEW QUESTIONS

1. Define cognitive strategies and explain how they can be used during exercise.

2. What is the difference between associating and dissociating during exercise?

3. Explain how and when you should associate during CRE activity?

4. Explain how and when you should dissociate during CRE activity?

5. Explain how and when you should associate during muscular fitness activity?

6. Explain how and when you should dissociate during muscular fitness activity?

7. Explain how and when you should associate during flexibility activity?

8. Explain how and when you should dissociate during flexibility activity?

9. What is positive self-talk and explain how you can use positive self-talk to increase the quality of your exercise experience.

10. Define imagery and list and explain three types of imagery skills.

11. Explain how you can incorporate imagery into your exercise program.

LAB ASSIGNMENT 11.1

Your assignment is to determine the effectiveness of using cognitive strategies on exercise performance, enjoyment, motivation, and commitment. Read the instructions below, answer the questions and have some fun!

Questions 1-3 should be answered before you begin exercising for the week.

1. Over the next two weeks, select 1or more exercise(s) for each component of health-related fitness that you will do at least two times per week. In the column below, list the exercise(s) that you plan to use to improve your health-related fitness over the next two weeks.

CRE				
MF				
Flexibility				

2. Prior to using your cognitive strategies, rank your overall level of enjoyment, motivation, and commitment to exercise in each area of health-related fitness from 1 (extremely low) to 9 (extremely high).

Enjoyment

CRE	1 2 3 4 5 6 7 8 9
MF	1 2 3 4 5 6 7 8 9
Flexibility	1 2 3 4 5 6 7 8 9

Motivation

CRE	1 2 3 4 5 6 7 8 9
MF	1 2 3 4 5 6 7 8 9
Flexibility	1 2 3 4 5 6 7 8 9

Commitment

CRE	1 2 3 4 5 6 7 8 9
MF	1 2 3 4 5 6 7 8 9
Flexibility	1 2 3 4 5 6 7 8 9

3. Over the next two weeks, select 1 associative and 1 dissociative strategy that you will use during your exercise workouts. List the strategies and explain why you selected each?

	Associative Strategy	Disassociative Strategy
CRE	1.	1.
MF	1.	1.
Flexibility	1.	1.

Questions 4-11 should be answered after you have completed your two weeks of exercising.

4. Rank your overall level of enjoyment, motivation, and commitment to exercise in each area of health-related fitness from 1 (extremely low) to 9 (extremely high).

Enjoyment

CRE	1	2	3	4	5	6	7	8	9
MF	1	2	3	4	5	6	7	8	9
Flexibility	1	2	3	4	5	6	7	8	9

Motivation

CRE	1	2	3	4	5	6	7	8	9
MF	1	2	3	4	5	6	7	8	9
Flexibility	1	2	3	4	5	6	7	8	9

Commitment

CRE	1	2	3	4	5	6	7	8	9
MF	1	2	3	4	5	6	7	8	9
Flexibility	1	2	3	4	5	6	7	8	9

5. Circle the cognitive strategy you enjoyed the most for CRE, MF, and Flexibility and explain why you like it more than the other strategy?

    CRE   Association   Dissociation
    MF   Association   Dissociation
    Flexibility   Association   Dissociation

6. Is there a strategy that you disliked? If so, for which exercise and explain why?

7. Which strategy increased your motivation to work on improving your CRE, MF, and Flexibility? Circle all that apply.

    Association   Dissociation   Both   Neither

8. Which strategy increased your level of commitment to work on improving your CRE, MF, and/or flexibility? Circle all that apply.

    Association   Dissociation   Both   Neither

9. Which strategy improved your performance more in your CRE, MF, and flexibility workouts? Circle all that apply.

CRE	Association	Dissociation	Both	Neither
MF	Association	Dissociation	Both	Neither
Flexibility	Association	Dissociation	Both	Neither

10. Discuss the overall success you had in implementing association and dissociation into your exercises.

11. Do you plan on using association and/or dissociation as part of your exercise program in the future? Please explain.

Association/Dissociation	CRE Exercises	YES	NO
Association/Dissociation	Muscular Fitness Exercises	YES	NO
Association/Dissociation	Flexibility Exercises	YES	NO

LAB ASSIGNMENT 11.2

Using Positive Self Talk to Increase Your Motivation to Exercise

1. Identify any components of health-related fitness that you have negative thoughts about and lack motivated to work on even though you know you should.

2. Using the "Transforming Negative Self-Talk Into Positive Self-Talk" chart located in Appendix A list your negative thoughts.

3. Explain why you lack motivation to improve your fitness in these area(s).

4. Over the next week, you are invited to begin using positive self-talk with the areas(s) of fitness listed in Q1.

a. Using positive self-talk, convert the negative statements into positive cues or triggers (e.g., I can do it; I am doing great! Reach my goal! 1 more!) and list them next to your negative statements on your Appendix A chart.. Make a few copies to put in your exercise bag, attach to your workout cards, use as a screen saver, tape to your desk or place on your wall.

5. For the next week, plan to use these positive statements in your workouts. In fact, you can even set a goal to use a certain number of positive statements in your workout.

6. When the week is up, answer the following:
   a. I enjoyed using positive self-talk while exercising

1	2	3	4	5	6	7	8	9

   not at all   somewhat   very much

   b. Positive self-talk motivated me to want to exercise more

1	2	3	4	5	6	7	8	9

   not at all   somewhat   very much

   c. Positive self-talk increased my commitment to make exercise a part of my life.

1	2	3	4	5	6	7	8	9

   not at all   somewhat   very much

   d. Positive self-talk enhanced my exercise performance

1	2	3	4	5	6	7	8	9

   not at all   somewhat   very much

LAB ASSIGNMENT 11.3

Using Imagery to Enhance Your Exercise Experiences

Answer questions 1-3 before you use imagery with your exercise(s).

1. Take a few minutes and think about what you would like to image either before, during, or after you exercise.

2. Write down your imagery scenario and read it over a few times so you can experience the positive feelings and emotions that you would want to receive from exercising.

3. For the next week, select a time when you will use imagery either before, during, or after your exercises and fill in the following:
   a. I will use imagery   before   during   after   I exercise.

Questions 4-8 should be answered after you have completed imagery and have exercised.

4. I used imagery   before my exercise   during my exercise   after my exercise

5. Evaluate your success incorporating the three Imagery elements.

   Vividness | 1 | 2 | 3 | 4 | 5 | 6 | 7 | 8 | 9 |
   |---|---|---|---|---|---|---|---|---|

                   poor   average   excellent

Controllability	1	2	3	4	5	6	7	8	9
	poor				average				excellent

Sensory Awareness	1	2	3	4	5	6	7	8	9
	poor				average				excellent

6. Explain any problems you had with imagery.

7. Circle the number that best describes your experience using imagery with your exercises

   a. I enjoyed using imagery with exercise

1	2	3	4	5	6	7	8	9
not at all				somewhat				very much

   b. Imagery motivated me to want to exercise more

1	2	3	4	5	6	7	8	9
not at all				somewhat				very much

   c. Imagery increased my commitment to make exercise a part of my life.

1	2	3	4	5	6	7	8	9
not at all				somewhat				very much

   d. Imagery increased my exercise performance

1	2	3	4	5	6	7	8	9
not at all				somewhat				very much

   e. I will make imagery part of my exercise routine.

1	2	3	4	5	6	7	8	9
definitely not				maybe				definitely so

8. Which of the four cognitive strategies did you enjoy most and least and explain why?

9. Six months from now, which cognitive strategies can you see yourself using with your exercise? Circle all that apply and explain your answer..

   Association   Dissociation   Positive Self-Talk   Imagery

10. Which of the cognitive strategies would you recommend to a friend and why

REFERENCES AND RECOMMENDED READINGS

Couture, R.T., Jerome, W., & Tihanyi, J. (1999). Can associative and dissociative strategies affect swimming performance of recreational swimmers? *The Sport Psychologist*, *13*, 334-343.

Martin, J., Dubbert, P.M., Katell, A.D., Thompson, J.K., Raczynski, J.R., Lake, M.,Smith, P.O. Webster, J.S., Sikora, T., & Cohen, R.E. (1984). The behavioral control of exercise in sedentary adults: Studies 1 through 6. *Journal of Consulting and ClinicalPsychology, 52, 795-811.*

Masters, K.S. & Olges, B.M. (1998a). Associative and dissociative cognitive strategies in exercise and running: 20 years later, what do we know. *The Sport Psychologist*, *12,* 253-270.

Mikes, J. (1987). Basketball fundamentals. A complete mental training guide. Champaign, Il: Leisure Press.

Morgan, W.P., & Pollack, M.L. (1977). Psychological characterization of the elite distance runner. *Annals of the New York Academy of Sciences*, *301,* 382-403.

Nietfeld, J.L. (2003). An examination of metacognitive strategy use and monitoring skills by competitive middle distance runners. *Journal of Applied Sport Psychology,* **15,** 307-320.

Scott, M.L., Scott, D., Bedic, S.P., & Dowd, J. (1999).The effect of associative and dissociative strategies on rowing ergometer performance. *The Sport Psychologist*, *13,* 57-68.

Vealy, R.S., & Greenleaf, C.A. (2006). Seeing is believing: Understanding and using imagery in sport. In J. M. Williams, Applied sport psychology: Personal growth to peak performance, 5th edition, pp 306-307.

Weinberg, R.S., & D. Gould. (2003). Exercise behavior and adherence. In Weinberg, R.S. & Gould, D. *Foundations of Sport and Exercise Psychology*, 3rd edition, pp 418-419. Human Kinetics: Champaign, IL.

Weinberg, R.S. & Gould, D. (2003). Self-talk. In Weinberg, R.S. & Gould, D. *Foundations of sport and exercise psychology*, 3rd edition, pp 364-367. Human Kinetics: Champaign, IL.

APPENDIX A
TRANSFORMING NEGATIVE SELF-TALK INTO POSITIVE SELF-TALK

My Negative Thoughts	My Newly Transformed Positive Thoughts

Chapter 12

Managing Your Stress

OVERVIEW

In this chapter you will:

- Learn what stress is
- Identify stressors in you life
- Discover how to take control of your stress
- Incorporate stress management techniques into your daily life
- Determine how exercise transforms negative stress into positive stress

At some point in our lives, we have all experienced a great deal of stress. In fact, many of us are surrounded by stress on a daily basis trying to tackle some of the following: (1) doing well and being productive in school and/or work; (2) taking care of finances; (3) managing our time effectively; (4) building positive relationships; (5) fulfilling family obligations; and (6) trying to take better care of ourselves;

Approximately two-thirds of adults experience large amounts of stress at least 1 day a week and it is estimated that it costs the United States government and businesses between 30 and 44 billion dollars annually for the treatment and consequences of stress and stress-related illness, (health care costs; worker absenteeism; reduction in job productivity) (International Labour Organization, 2000). The simple fact is that stress is everywhere (Blonna, 2005). Whether in school (adjusting to a new living environment, dealing with academic pressure, meeting new people), at home (balancing relationship demands, family and financial responsibilities), at work (succeeding at work, getting along with peers, handling the pressure of job responsibilities), playing sports (pressure to win; dealing with losing) or exercising (uncertainty of using equipment properly, being uncomfortable around others, not seeing results, feeling guilty if you miss a workout), you will find stress. And if you don't find stress, then stress with find you.

Your commitment to first identify the cause of your stress and then choose how to handle it will ultimately determine how successful you are in managing your stress effectively and minimizing the frequency of highly stressful experiences. In this chapter, you will learn what stress is and how to deal with it effectively in your lives. In addition, you will learn a variety of coping strategies designed to transform negative stress into positive stress. Finally, you will learn how to take control of your stress and empower yourself to live your life the way you want to rather than have to.

WHAT IS STRESS?

Over the years, there has been a considerable amount of work done in the area of stress and stress and management. Consequently, a number of popular definitions are currently being used to define and understand what stress is. For example, renowned researcher Robert Lazarus defined stress as a state of anxiety produced when events and responsibilities exceed one's coping abilities (Lazuras & DeLongis, 1983). McGrath (1970) defined stress as a substantial imbalance between psychological and/or physical demand and response capability, under where failure to meet that demand has important consequences. Perhaps the most popular definition of stress comes from Hans Selye, one of the leading authorities on stress who defined stress as a nonspecific response of the body to any demand placed upon it (Selye, 1976). In essence, any time the body reacts to a demand (e.g., exercise overload, job promotion, family argument) you are under stress. One final way to define stress is to view it as the result of imbalance between life's demands and one's ability to handle these demands. For example, when you never seem to have enough time to do what you want to do or when your mind is racing with ideas and you just cannot seem to get your thoughts straight there is an imbalance between life's demands and your ability to handle them thus creating stress.

What Causes Stress?

Any fact or situation, event or circumstance, feedback or stimulus that is perceived to be a threat is known as a stressor or that which causes or promotes stress. Stressors can be identified by time and how long they last. For example, acute stressors are often the result of a rapid-onset of stress which pops up unexpectedly (e.g., hearing a loud noise late at night while you were sleeping) and then goes away. Chronic stressors are long lasting and usually unassociated with an immediate warning (e.g., loud noise), which causes physiological arousal to last for extended periods of time (days, weeks, months, years) For example, Joyce is a woman who worries on a daily basis regardless of any new events occurring in her life. She worries about getting her children off to school on time, making sure the house is clean, getting to work on time and being productive, making dinner that her family likes, helping her husband with his career and spending quality time with her family. Even though she has a set routine and successfully completes it all, it does not stop Joyce from feeling stressed on a daily basis. Consequently, Joyce's life appears to be one big chronic stress.

Sources of Stressors

Stressors can come from a variety of sources that people encounter in their lives and they include:

- *physical stressors*—which happen when the body is overloaded resulting in tension, discomfort or pain in one or more parts of the body (e.g., muscles, joints, etc);
- *psychological stressors*—occur when the mind is preoccupied with thoughts of worry, nervousness, apprehension or there is a threat to one's self-esteem;
- *social stressors*—are when people feel uncomfortable in crowds and/or have difficulty being around others;
- *environmental stressors*— are related to air pollution, noise, weather and temperature that are known to affect one's mood, attitude, and the amount of stress perceived on a daily basis;
- *biochemical stressors*—are related to the changes that the body undergoes resulting from air pollution, temperature, humidity, nutrition, drugs, and alcohol;
- *nutritional stressors*—has to do with our eating patterns; when we eat poorly (e.g., overeat, eat the wrong foods, skip meals) we may become nutrient deficient causing the body to be missing what it needs to function efficiently, resulting in the body having to overwork itself to perform normal daily functions;
- *academic stressors*—can result from having difficulty in school (e.g., not enjoying classes, poor communication with instructors and administrators, difficulty understanding coursework; can't find a major of interest; being overloaded with exams, etc);
- *philosophical stressors*—occur when you have a lack of purpose or direction in life (e.g. not knowing what you want out of life, uncertainty about what to major in college, being in the wrong job or career or questioning whether you are going in the right direction);

STRESS AND THE STRESS PROCESS

After being confronted with stress, people exhibit a certain behavioral pattern known as stress reactivity (see Figure 12.1 for a list of reactions people have when confronted by stressors) or the way you react to stressors. It was Walter Cannon, a Harvard University physiologist who in the early 1900's was the first to explain how people react to stress as the fight-or-flight-response. According to Cannon, when people are faced with stress, they have two choices: (1) stand up and confront the stress = "fight it" or (2) run away from it = "flight" (Cannon, 1922).

Picture this: Adam is upset with his boss (Mindy) for not getting the promotion he was promised. Each time he sees Mindy, Adam wants to convey his feelings (fight) only to be stopped by his stress (flight). He is concerned, however, that if he does not speak with Mindy (fight), his anger will get the best of him and cause him to overact. Consequently, Adam has kept his emotions inside of himself (flight) leaving him with a very important choice: speak with Mindy and let her know how he feels (fight) or avoid talking to her about his upset and keep it inside (flight). After careful consideration, Adam decides to talk with Mindy, recognizing that the only way he could truly get rid of his stress was to talk with Mindy and let her know how he felt about not getting promoted. While Adam may have no choice in Mindy's final decision, he does have a choice in the way he chooses to deal with his stress (fight or flight). Speaking with Mindy clearly gives Adam the opportunity to take control of his stress.

1. Elevated heart rate	8. Shortness of breath
2. Rapid breathing	9. Fatigue
3. Diarrhea	10. Headaches
4. Constipation	11. Dizziness
5. Dry mouth	12. Sleep disturbances
6. Low back pain	13. Memory problems
7. Irritability and moodiness	14. Lack of concentration

Figure 12.1—Reactions to Stress

It is important to note that neither "flight or "fight" is necessarily any better or worse than the other. In some instances, you may be better off standing your ground and take action (fight) while other times you may be better off looking the other way (fight) and not letting stress get the best of you by acting inappropriately. It really depends on you, the stressors you are dealing with and the situation(s) that you are in.

GENERAL ADAPTATION SYNDROME (GAS)

Developed by Selye, GAS is a three-stage process that explains how people react to stress: (1) alarm; (2) resistance; (3) exhaustion (Selye, 1974)).

Alarm Phase—As you perceive a stressor(s), your body's balance becomes disturbed and prepares itself for sudden action. For example, you are sleeping in your bed late at night and you hear a loud noise. Immediately, your senses become sharpened resulting in several physiological changes (e.g., heart starts to beat faster; respiration, blood pressure, perspiration, and muscular tension increases).

Resistance Phase—Here, your body attempts to adjust to your stressor(s) and return back to its normal physiological balance known as homeostasis. Your heart rate, respiration, blood pressure, perspiration and muscular tension all begin to decrease as you prepare to make decisions about how to handle your stress (e.g., turn the alarm off). However, if stress continues and you cannot adapt to it, you will enter the third and final phase.

Exhaustion Phase—Your endocrine system cannot produce a sufficient amount of hormones to counter the chronic stressors you are dealing with. If this continues over long periods of time (weeks, months or even years), it can affect your heart, blood pressure, stomach, muscles and joints causing headaches, fatigue, dizziness, cramping, and other more serious debilitating conditions (e.g., heart disease).

Example: Morris comes home from a long day at school and decides he is going to catch up on some sleep. As he gets ready to take a nap, he realizes that he has an important paper due tomorrow that he has not started yet. Immediately, his bodily functions begin to change as he experiences increases in muscular tension and heart rate (alarm phase). In order to counter these feelings, Morris decides to sit down for an hour and start writing his paper. Upon doing so, Morris has redirected his focus from being stressed about forgetting his paper to getting it done (resistance phase). Consequently, he has successfully resisted his stress and now feels better. However, if at any point Morris thinks he will never finish his paper or becomes upset with himself for leaving it for the last minute, his stress will increase and cause possible exhaustion especially if this type of behavior lingers on.

TAKING RESPONSIBILITY AND CONTROL OF YOUR STRESS

In life, there are many things that can cause you stress. For example, losing your job, failing an exam, mourning the loss of a loved one or having a fight with a significant other can certainly cause stress for you. However, what determines whether your stress goes away or lingers on in your life is how you choose to deal with it. Will you take responsibility for your stress and gain control over it or will you attempt to push it away and blame others, find excuses, or pretend everything is ok when you know it is not? (See Figure 12.2 for a list of perceived causes of stress).

Family	School	Work	Friends	Finances
Parents	Teachers	Bosses	Relationships	Money
Siblings	Classmates	Co-workers		Salary
Other family members	Courses	Salary		Bills
	Homework	Benefits		
		Responsibilities		

Figure 12.2—Perceived Causes of Stress

All too often, people look to blame others for their stressors and neglect to take full responsibility for their actions or interpretations. Phrases like: "It's your fault that I... If only you would have... You make me so upset... It's not fair that you got... I did it because you... are prime examples of how we attempt to redirect our stress by justifying its causes through the blaming and making up of reasons for our actions. If only it was that easy. Just blame someone else every time things do not go your way and you get upset. The problem is that when you do that, you wind up retaining the stress. In fact, it is rather common for people to experience high levels of stress simply by thinking about someone whom they have had disagreements with, became upset with or argued with in the past (even when these people are not around you).

Unfortunately, blaming others for your stress or justifying how things are unfair when situations or opportunities do not go your way is not going to take the stress away. In fact, your stress level will only increase. For example, take Brady and Keisha, a happily married couple who get into an argument resulting in each of them getting very angry and barking profanities at each other. Their choices are to take responsibility for what they said and/or did or blame the other for their stress-provoking actions. Doing the former will most likely lead to a reduction and possible elimination of stress because they both recognized that their causes of stress came from themselves and not the other, thus giving them the freedom to choose how to handle their stress.

Conversely, blaming each other for their stress and neglecting to take full responsibility for their actions will only result in increasing their stress because their perceived stressors (what they think to be causing their stress) are not within their control. So while Brady cannot control what Keisha said and vice versa, each can control the way they interpret what was said. They can choose to react in rage or anger or apologize for the other being upset. They can choose to blame the other for their stress or walk away from the situation before losing control. Finally, they can stop talking to each other and keep the stress inside or they can let each other know that they were upset with what was said to them.

To put it simply, if you cannot control your stressor, then do not waste time thinking about it. Taking control of your stress means that you perceive yourself to be the cause of your stress response and once you recognize that the way you handle your stress is 100% within your control, you are on your way towards living a healthier, stress-free lifestyle (most of the time). Below is a list of five common, potentially stressful situations that identify what you are and are not in control of in order to reduce your stress.

1. ***Relationships***—You have an argument with a significant other and you are hurt by what was said to you. Although you cannot control what your significant other said, you can control the way you perceive what was said. Do you let it bother you or do you look to rid yourself of the stress?

2. ***School***—You are stressed in one of your classes because of all the work that has to be done. Perhaps you are unhappy with your grade or you are not getting along with your instructor. While you cannot control the amount of coursework given in class,

you can control how much time you study and whether you choose to ask your teacher questions in the event that you do not understand something. In addition, you cannot control the grade being given, but you can decide whether to speak with your teacher about your grade and why you think you deserve better.

3. *Work*—Sometimes you may become stressed at work because you do not like the way your boss is treating you, the work that you do or the environment that you spend a significant amount of time in. What you cannot control is your boss' behavior. However, what you can control is how you interpret what your boss says. You can choose to speak with your boss and let him/her know how you feel rather than keep it all inside of you. You can also choose to quit your job and find something else. In time, you will realize that when you take a proactive stand to get rid of your stressors by choosing to do something about it (e.g., fight), rather than adopting a defeatist attitude that there is nothing you can do, the stress that appears to surround you begins to disappear and you become empowered in your life.

4. *Finances*—You may be stressed because you do not have enough money and you may even be faced with financial debt (student loans, rent, mortgage, taxes, car payments). It is important to note that you are the one who controls how much money you make as well as how much money you spend. Granted, times are tough for many people. Presently, the cost of living has exceeded the annual raises that people are getting in many popular professions (e.g., teaching) resulting in what once may have been affordable, now becoming too costly. Choosing to take control over your finances means that you will figure a way to earn more money and/or spend money more efficiently.

5. *Time management*—Finally, how about investigating your time management skills? Do you ever feel like there is never enough time to do what you want to do? No matter how much you accomplish in any given day, there is always more to do the next day? Well, how much time do you make to procrastinate (e.g., watch television, play video games, talk on your cell phone, interact on facebook or twitter)? There are 24 hours, 1440 minutes and 86,400 seconds in every day. While some days may indeed be busier than others, everyone has at least a few minutes each and every day to find the time to accomplish what they set out to do. In fact, when you believe that you would be doing more things that you want to (e.g., exercising, eating healthier) if you only had the "time" you are really making a choice to do other things with your time. Imagine if you planned to take a few minutes out of your day to do something because you wanted to and not because you thought you had to. Your stress would decrease and you would probably accomplish more in that day that you usually do. In lab 12.6 you will learn how to decrease your stress by managing your time more effectively.

So anytime you find yourself blaming others for your stress and resenting the fact that this is happening to you, take a step back and gain control. Decide what you can do to get rid of your stress and do it. And remember, if the stressor is out of your control and there is nothing you can do to get rid of it then let go of it and move on.

REDUCING YOUR STRESS

Just because you have identified your stressors and learned whether or not they are within your control, that does not mean you will never become stressed. Face it, stress is an everyday part of our lives. The more you know about the causes of your stress, your reactions to your stressors and how to deal with your stress the more success you will have in reducing and eventually eliminating many of your life's stressors. There are a variety of stress management techniques that you can use to reduce your stress. In this section, you will be introduced to five of the most popular and effective: (1) progressive muscle relaxation; (2) relaxation response; (3) yogic breathing; (4) time out; and (5) exercise. Each one is uniquely designed to help transform negative stress into positive stress. So grab your stress and be prepared to get rid of it!

Progressive Muscle Relaxation (PMR) was developed by Edmund Jacobson in the 1930's and teaches you how to distinguish muscular tension from muscular relaxation, thus making you more sensitive to how your body feels when you become stressed. Unfortunately, people sometimes do not realize they are under physical stress until they are in pain (e.g., back aches after sitting arched behind your desk for hours at a time; muscular cramps after putting too much stress on the body; stomach aches after overeating). PMR heightens your awareness to become more receptive to muscular tension before actually feeling pain by becoming more aware of the physiological messages received from your body (e.g., slight muscle aches, body discomfort). PMR can be done for short (a few minutes) or long (thirty minutes or more) periods of time as well as in a variety of locations (at your desk, in your car, on the train, in the lunchroom, in your bed, at the gym, in fact, almost anywhere). PMR is recommended for people who experience stress physically before mentally. Common symptoms that generally let you know that you are under physical stress include muscle aches and pains, cramping, gastrointestinal problems, headaches, nausea. See figure 12.3 for instructions on how to use PMR.

Relaxation Response (RR)—was developed by Herbert Benson (1975) and emphasizes a state of deep rest that includes the following four components:

1. a quiet environment—select a place that is free from noise or distractions that allows you to focus on yourself without being interrupted;

2. a passive attitude—allow your thoughts to enter and exit your mind without analyzing, evaluating, criticizing or questioning; avoid over-thinking; in time, these thoughts will learn to disappear just as quickly as they appear;

1. Start out by selecting the order of body parts you want to begin tensing and relaxing first. It is recommended that you start all the way at the bottom (toes) or top (head) and continue in a straight line until all major muscle groups have been tensed and relaxed (e.g., forehead, eyebrows, cheeks, neck, shoulders, chest, back, triceps, biceps, wrists, fingers, abdomen, buttocks quadriceps, hamstrings, calves, hip flexors, groin, shins, ankles, toes).

2. Inhale through your nose and hold your breath as you tighten up identified muscles for 3-5 seconds.

3. Exhale and relax identified muscle for 3-5 seconds.

4. Repeat process 2-5×.

5. Inhale and allow muscle group to relax (do not tighten up).

6. Exhale and keep muscle group relaxed.

7. Repeat process 2-5×.

8. Notice the difference in how relax that muscle group. (See lab 12.1 for a more detailed description of PMR).

Figure 12.3—Progressive Muscle Relaxation

3. a comfortable position—select a position that you feel comfortable and can stay in for at least 20 minutes without having to move around too much; the key is to feel comfortable, but not so comfortable that you will fall asleep;

4. a mantra—choose a word that you can repeat over and over again (either verbally or nonverbally) that creates a feeling of relaxation; For example, say you pick the word "relax" and begin to repeat "relax" to yourself. As time goes by, the word "relax" will enter your mind and push out thoughts that you do not want to think about (e.g., I have so much to do today; I am so tired). Once your mantra has kicked out your unwanted "stress provoking" thoughts, you are now to free to allow you mind to wander freely and explore places that create an immediate sense of freedom, tranquility and total mind-body relaxation.

RR is recommended for individuals who experience mental stress (worry, over-thinking) before physical stress. For example, Deb is someone who is constantly on the go thinking about all the things she has to do in a day. No matter how much work she gets done in a day, there is always more work for Deb to do. Even when she is physically drained, her mind is always working, thinking of what has to be done next, evaluating how the previous task was done, etc. What Deb needs is to take control of her thoughts and RR is one way to do that. With a little practice, Deb can learn to use her "mantra" in situations where she feels her thoughts are counterproductive and causing her undue stress. She can also use RR as a way to cleanse and refresh her mind and body after a long, hard day. See Lab 12.2 to familiarize yourself with RR.

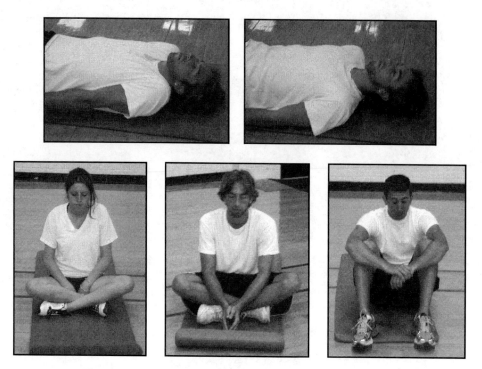

Figure 12.4—Progressive Muscle Relaxation and Response

Yogic Breathing—involves manipulating your breathing pattern so that you eventually learn how to control your breathing response; Yogic breathing works on a 1:4:2 count which begins with an inhalation of 4 seconds, followed by holding your breath for 16 seconds and completed by exhaling for 8 seconds. Typically, when someone is stressed their breathing pattern is labored resulting in rapid inhaling and exhaling leading to possible shortness of breath. Through yogic breathing, you will become more sensitive to your normal breathing pattern and in times of stress, your awareness of your breathing will be heightened, thus helping you to concentrate and eventually control your breathing pattern. This will inevitably take your mind off of your stressors and allow you to feel more relaxed. See lab 12.3 to learn more about using yogic breathing to reduce your stress.

Time Out—In times where you recognize that you are under high levels of stress that just won't go away, one of the best strategies for you to employ is to remove yourself from that stressful environment and take a "time out." For example, in sport, when a coach sees his team playing poorly and not performing up to their potential, he/she calls a time out to stop things from getting worse. In your case, you are calling a time out to stop your stress from increasing. Simply remove yourself from your stressful situation and go someplace else. By walking away you are stopping yourself from fighting a losing battle and giving yourself an opportunity to redirect your thoughts, channel your energy and empower yourself towards overcoming your stressors and feeling better.

Exercise—Last, but certainly not least is exercise. Over the years, research has indicated that exercise is successful in reducing stress across a variety of populations (e.g., college students, fit vs. unfit individuals, spinal cord injury patients), (Berger & Owen, 1988, Berger, Friedman, & Eaton, 1988; Crews & Landers, 1987, Latimer, et al., 2004). As you exercise, you begin to place more than the usual amount of physical stress on the body (overload) which can redirect you from distress (negative stress) to eustress (positive stress) and invigorate the mind and body to feel better. Researchers have hypothesized that during exercise, the body releases endorphins which are a morphine-like substance that act as natural painkillers, creating a euphoric like state of well-being. Exercise is also known to create a distraction from daily stressors by forcing you to concentrate (at least some of the time) on important exercise information (e.g., heart rate, breathing pattern, muscular tension, proper form, equipment). Most important, once you begin to see and feel improvements from exercise your self-esteem may increase and you will begin to look at exercise as something positive and worthwhile, especially under times of stress. Think about it for a moment. You are under a lot of stress and you decide to go exercise to get rid of it. Right away, that should make you feel better because you are taking control of your stress. Rather than letting it get worse or blame others for your stress, you simply recognized that you did not want to feel stressed and decided to go exercise.

In conclusion, stress is something that is part of everyone's lives. However, the amount of stress we encounter on a daily basis and the way we choose to handle our stress is totally up to us. Learning how to take responsibility for our stressors and control the way we react to them is a power way to live life. So the next time you are under stress, I invite you to ask yourself, "Who's in control?" Then powerfully look in the mirror and respond, "I am." Then choose any of the stress management techniques mentioned in this chapter and be proud of yourself for the decisions you made and all that you have accomplished.

REVIEW QUESTIONS

1. Define stress. Explain what stress means to you.

2. What causes stress?

3. List three to five sources of stress and describe how each exists in your life.

4. Define the "Fight vs. Flight" response and give an example of how you have used each in your life.

5. What is the General Adaptation Syndrome?

6. Explain the difference between taking control of your stressors and letting stress control you.

7. Identify a situation in your life where you have not taken responsibility for your stress. What were the results?

8. What will you do over the next week to take responsibility for the stress that you are presently experiencing in your life?

9. Discuss several ways that you have learned to take control of your stress.

10. List at least three different stress management techniques and explain how to use each.

LAB ASSIGNMENT 12.1
TAKING CONTROL OF YOUR STRESS

Answer the following:

1. Stress occurs in my life when _____

    _____

    _____

2. Identify one stressful situation that occurred in your life this week.

3. Explain the causes(s) of your stress?

4. Are you in control of the stress that occurred in your life the last week?
    YES   NO   NOT SURE

5. If you are in control of your stress, what do you do to stay in control?

6. If you are not in control of your stress, discuss why you are choosing to focus on it and how does this make you feel?

7. Explain your coping skills for dealing with the stress you identified above. Did you reduce your stress? Explain why or why not?

LAB ASSIGNMENT 12.2
TRANSFORMING STRESS INTO SUCCESS

1. Identify one successful and one unsuccessful experience that occurred in your life.

   Successful experience _____

   _____

   _____

   Unsuccessful experience _____

   _____

   _____

2. Explain the differences in your perceptions and behaviors for each experience.

3. For your successful experience—List three strengths that helped you to achieve success

4. For your unsuccessful experience—List three barriers that stopped you from being more successful.

5. Is it within your control to live a successful life? If so explain how and if not, explain what is presently stopping you.

6. Over the next week, your assignment is to create one successful experience that you want to happen. What strengths will you utilize to create success? What strategies will you incorporate in the event you get stopped?

7. In order for me to succeed this week, I will _____

   _____

   _____

   and I will not _____

   _____

   _____

After the week is up, answer the following:

8. Were you successful? Explain why or why not.

9. How did this experience affect the level of stress in your life (e.g., increase, decrease, stayed the same).

10. What did you enjoy more—seeking success and focusing on the process or being successful (outcome)?

11. Can you see yourself seeking success on a daily basis? If so, write down what you will succeed at next week. If not, write down what is stopping you and what and when you plan to do to get rid of it.

LAB ASSIGNMENTS 12.3, 12.4, 12.5, 12.6, AND 12.7
INCORPORATING STRESS MANAGEMENT TECHNIQUES
INTO YOUR LIFESTYLE

Over the next few weeks plan to practice each of the following five stress management techniques:

(1) Progressive Muscle Relaxation (PMR)

(2) Relaxation Response (RR)

(3) Yogic Breathing

(4) Taking Control of Your Time

(5) Exercise

Lab Questions are listed separately for each of the five Stress Management Techniques in labs 12.3 (PMR), 12.4 (RR), 12.5 (Yogic Breathing), 12.6 (Taking Control of Your Time) and 12.7 (Exercise) as well as collectively in lab assignment 12.8.

LAB ASSIGNMENT 12.3
PROGRESSIVE MUSCLE RELAXATION

Over the next week, select a day and time that you are committed to practicing Progressive Muscle Relaxation (PMR) and jot it down in the space below.

I will practice PMR on _____, the _____ day of _____ at _____ AM/PM at _____ (name of place).

Here is an example of PMR starting with the toes and finishing with the eyebrows

• inhale for 3-5 seconds and tighten the toes on your left foot

• exhale for 3-5 seconds and relax the toes on your left foot

- inhale for 3-5 seconds and tighten the toes on your right foot
- exhale for 3-5 seconds and relax the toes on your right foot
- inhale for 3-5 seconds and tighten your left ankle
- exhale for 3-5 seconds and relax your left ankle
- inhale for 3-5 seconds and tighten your right ankle
- exhale for 3-5 seconds and relax your right ankle
- inhale for 3-5 seconds and tighten your left hamstring
- exhale for 3-5 seconds and relax your left hamstring
- inhale for 3-5 seconds and tighten your right hamstring
- exhale for 3-5 seconds and relax your right hamstring
- inhale for 3-5 seconds and tighten your left quadricep
- exhale for 3-5 seconds and relax your left quadricep
- inhale for 3-5 seconds and tighten your right quadricep
- exhale for 3-5 seconds and relax your right quadricep
- inhale for 3-5 seconds and expand abdomen up to the ceiling
- exhale for 3-5 seconds and relax you abdomen
- inhale for 3-5 seconds and expand chest up to the ceiling
- exhale for 3-5 seconds and relax your chest
- inhale for 3-5 seconds and raise your shoulders up to your neck
- exhale for 3-5 seconds and relax your shoulders
- inhale for 3-5 seconds and make a tight fist with your left hand
- as you exhale let one finger at a time go starting with the thumb-index-middle-ring and pinky
- inhale for 3-5 seconds and make a tight fist with your right hand
- as you exhale let one finger at a time go starting with the thumb-index-middle-ring-and pinky
- inhale for 3-5 seconds and turn neck your as far to the left as you can
- exhale for 3-5 seconds and allow your neck to return to the center of your body
- inhale for 3-5 seconds and turn your neck all the way to the right
- exhale for 3-5 seconds and allow your neck to return to its normal resting place
- inhale for 3-5 seconds as you touch your chin to your chest
- exhale for 3-5 seconds and allow your chin to return to its normal resting place
- inhale for 3-5 seconds as you tilt your head all the back
- exhale for 3-5 seconds as you allow your head to return back to its normal resting place
- inhale for 3-5 seconds as you smile as wide as you can
- exhale for 3-5 seconds as you let your face relax

- inhale for 3-5 seconds as you raise your eyebrows to the top of your head
- exhale for 3-5 seconds as your allow your eyebrows to descend back to its normal resting place
- take all the tension in the body and transform it into your hands by rubbing them briskly back and forth until you feel heat; then place your palms gently over your eyelids; the warm sensation you are experiencing represents a transformation from physical stress to relaxation;

After completing your PMR exercise answer the following:

1. Who invented PMR?

2. What is the correct procedure for using PMR?

3. What did you like about PMR?

4. How did PMR affect your level of stress?

5. Can you see yourself using PMR to reduce your stress on a weekly basis?

6. If yes, list two different times and places that you will consider incorporating PMR into your life?

7. If no, explain what you disliked about PMR?

LAB ASSIGNMENT 12.4
RELAXATION RESPONSE

Over the next week, select a day and time that you are committed to practicing Relaxation Response (RR) and jot it down in the space below.

I will practice PMR on _____, the _____ day of _____ at _____ AM/PM at _____ (name of place).

Once you have completed RR answer the following questions:

1. Who invented relaxation response (RR)?

2. Define the four components of RR?

3. What is the mantra that you used and did it work to take your mind off of your stress?

4. What did you like about RR?

5. How did RR affect your level of stress?

6. Can you see yourself using RR to reduce your stress on a weekly basis?

7. If yes, list two different times and places that you will consider incorporating RR into your life?

8. If no, explain what you disliked about RR?

LAB ASSIGNMENT 12.5
YOGIC BREATHING

Over the next week, select a day and time that you are committed to practicing Yogie Breathing and jot it down in the space below.

I will practice PMR on _____, the _____ day of _____ at _____ AM/PM at _____ (name of place).

Once you have completed yogic breathing, answer the following questions.

1. Define the proper breathing pattern for Yogic Breathing.

2. What did you like about Yogic Breathing?

3. How did Yogic Breathing affect your level of stress?

4. Can you see yourself using Yogic Breathing to reduce your stress on a weekly basis?

5. If yes, list two different times and places that you will consider incorporating Yogic Breathing into your life?

6. If no, explain what you disliked about Yogic Breathing?

LAB ASSIGNMENT 12.6
TAKING CONTROL OF YOUR TIME

The purpose of this assignment is for you to learn how to take control of your time and manage it successfully.

1. Over the next 24 hours, your time will be broken down into one-hour increments where you should record everything that you do in the column marked "Activity." Then in the column marked "Level of Stress Experienced", rank the stress that you have experienced from 1 (low) to 5 (moderate) to 9 (high) during that time period. In the third column, marked "How do you feel at this time?" record the thoughts that you are experiencing (e.g., happy, angry, energetic, sad, satisfied, etc) during this time period. If one day is not enough time for you to determine how you manage your time, you can repeat this exercise for as many consecutive days as you think you need to get a handle on your time management skills.

	Activity	Level of Stress Experienced	How do you feel at this time?
7 AM			
8 AM			
9 AM			
10 AM			
11 AM			
12 AM			
1 PM			
2 PM			
3 PM			
4 PM			
5 PM			
6 PM			
7 PM			
8 PM			
9 PM			
10 PM			
11 PM			
12 AM			
1 AM			
2 AM			
3 AM			
4 AM			
5 AM			
6 AM			

After completing the recording of your activities, answer the following.

2. What have you noticed about what you do with your time?

3. Explain how your time management skills play a role in the level of stress that you experience.

4. For the next week, organize yourself in the following manner. List all of the things you must do or get accomplished in the next day under Priority Column A. Then list all of the things that you would like to get accomplished, but can wait at least one day, but not more than three days under Priority Column B. Finally, in Priority Column C include all the things that you would like to accomplish, but can wait at least five or more days.

	Priority Column A Must Accomplish Today	Priority Column B Must Accomplish in Next 2-3 Days	Priority Column C Can Wait until Next Week
1.			
2.			
3.			
4.			
5.			
6.			
7.			
8.			

After the week is over, answer the following questions:

5. Place a check mark next to all of the items that you have listed and completed from your priority list in Q4.

6. Did you complete everything from your Priority A List?   YES   NO
    Explain why or why not?

7. If you answered "YES," explain how your stress has been affected by your accomplishments? If you answered "NO" explain what stopped you from accomplishing all of the items on Priority Lists A and B?

8. Explain how this exercise (writing down and ranking your list of priorities by importance) has helped you decrease your level of stress.

9. What do you have planned for next week?

10. What strategies will you incorporate to accomplish your agenda items on priority lists A and B.

LAB ASSIGNMENT 12.7
EXERCISE YOUR STRESS AWAY

1. Over the next week, select two days that will exercise and two days that you will not and jot down your schedule for each in the spaces listed below.

    Exercise Day 1 Time _____ Place _____ Activity _____

    Exercise Day 2 Time _____ Place _____ Activity _____

    No exercise   Date 1 _____ Date 2 _____

2. Prior to exercising answer the following:

    A. My mood is

1	2	3	4	5	6	7	8	9
Bad								Excellent

    B. My level of stress is

1	2	3	4	5	6	7	8	9
Low								High

    C. I am looking forward to exercising today

1	2	3	4	5	6	7	8	9
Not at All								Very Much

3. Write down the following as it pertains to your exercise workout:

    Activities you plan to do _____

    Time Committed to Exercising_____

    Place of Exercise_____

4. After completing your exercise answer the following:

   A. As a result of exercising my level of stress has

        INCREASED   DECREASED   REMAINED THE SAME

   B. My mood is

        BETTER   WORSE   THE SAME

   C. I have MORE LESS the SAME amount of energy now than before I started exercising

5. Explain the effect that exercise had on your level of stress.

6. Answer the following questions on the days that you did not exercise:

   A. My mood is

       1   2   3   4   5   6   7   8   9

       Bad   Excellent

   B. My level of stress is

       1   2   3   4   5   6   7   8   9

       Low   High

   C. I am looking forward to exercising today

       1   2   3   4   5   6   7   8   9

   Not at All   Very Much

7. What have you noticed about your level of stress on the days that you exercised vs. the days that you did not?

8. Do you plan to incorporate exercise into your life as a way to manage your stress? If so, explain when? If not, explain what is stopping you and what you plan to do to overcome your barriers?

LAB ASSIGNMENT 12.8

Now that you have practiced each of the five stress management techniques introduced in labs 10.3-10.7 let's see which ones are really for you.

1. Please rank the order of enjoyment for each of the five stress management techniques that you have been practicing for the past few weeks from 1 (did not enjoy) to 5 (enjoyed the most):

   Progressive Muscle Relaxation   _____

   Managing My Time Successfully   _____

   Relaxation Response   _____

   Exercise My Stress Away   _____

   Yogic Breathing   _____

2. Explain what you liked and/or disliked about each.

   Progressive Muscle Relaxation _____

   Relaxation Response _____

   Yogic Breathing _____

   Managing Time _____

   Exercise _____

3. What were your thoughts prior to and after practicing each technique?

4. Did you have any difficulties practicing any of these techniques? If so, list each.

5. Which of these techniques allowed you to feel 100% in control of your stress?

6. Five years from now, which techniques do you see as part of your lifestyle behavior and why?

REFERENCES AND RECOMMENDED READINGS

Benson, H. (1975). The relaxation response. New York: Avon Books

Berger, B.G., & Owen, D.R. (1988). Stress reduction and mood enhancement in four exercise modes: Swimming, body conditioning, Hatha yoga, and fencing. *Research Quarterly for Exercise and Sport,* 59, 148-159.

Berger, B., Friedman, E., & Eaton, M. (1988). Comparison of jogging, the Relaxation Response, and group interaction for stress reduction. *Journal of Sport & Exercise Psychology, 10*, 431-447.

Cannon, W. (1922). The wisdom of the body. New York: W.W. Norton.

Crews, D.J., & Landers, D.M. (1987). A meta-analytic review of aerobic fitness and reactivity to Psychosocial stressors. *Medicine and Science in Sports and Exercise, 19,* 114-120.

Inernational Labour Organization (2000). Press release Index: ILO report examines mental health in the workplace, in Finland, Germany, Poland, United Kingdom, United States, Costs of workplace stress are rising with depression increasingly common. October, 2000.

Jacobson, E. (1938). Progressive relaxation. 2nd edition. Chicago: University of Chicago Press.

Latimer, A.E., Martin Ginis, K.A., Hicks, A.L., & McCartney, N. (2004). An examination of the mechanisms of exercise-induced change in psychological well-being among people with spinal cord injury. *Journal of Rehabilitation Research & Development, 41*, 643-652.

Lazuras, R., & DeLongis, A. (1983). Psychological stress and coping in aging. *American Psychologist*, 38, 245-254.

Lox, C.L., Martin Ginis, K.A., & Petruzzello, S.J. (2006). The psychology of exercise: Integrating theory and practice, 2nd ed. pp 269-292, 346. Holcomb Hathaway: Scotsdale, AZ.

McGrath, J.E. (1970). Major methodological issues. In J.E. McGrath (Ed.), Social and psychological factors in stress (pp. 20). New York: Holt, Renehart, & Winston.

Selye, H. (1976). The stress of life. McGraw-Hill, New York.

Selye, H. (1974). Stress without distress. Lippincott, New York.